ENOUGH

OF

SUDDEN

DISEASES

AND

INFIRMITIES

TELLA OLAYERI

08023583168

Published By:

GOD'S LINK VENTURES

Email tellaolayeri@gmail.com

Website www.tellaolayeri.com

US Contact
Ruth Jack
14 Milewood Road
Verbank
N.Y.12585
U.S.A. +19176428989

APPRECIATION

I give special appreciation to my children and wife **MRS NGOZI OLAYERI** for her assistance in ensuring that this book is published.

Also, this manuscript wouldn't have seen light of the day, if not for the spiritual encouragement I gathered from my father in the Lord, **Dr. D. K. OLUKOYA** who served as spiritual mirror that brightens my hope to explore my calling (Evangelism)

We shall reap our blessings in heaven but the battle to make heaven is not over, until it is won.

PREFACE

In the world today, disease and sickness are claiming terrific toll of human lives. In spite of the fact that medical science is demonstrating its greatest achievements, disease advances in unprecedented measures all over the world.

Health is not negotiable. Life has no duplicate. It is insecure to toy with life, mostly when health is involved. Don't trade your life into the dustbin of life. Don't cut your destiny short. Call forth healings, vigour, vitality and hope for- good living.

Pray, so that you might not experience spiritual or physical sickness, financial sickness or boredom. Be prayerful, or else, your problems will stick on you, in as much you remain prayer less. This is the reason last chapter of this book is specifically dedicated to prayers. Pray the prayers and receive divine healing.

This book goes a long way to give both physical and spiritual solution to health problems. The book is systematically arranged to suit your needs. Above all, the treatments recommended in this book are intended as a reference volume. It is not intended as a substitute for any treatment prescribed by your doctor. The information

Here is design to help you make informed choices about your health. If you suspect that you have medical problem, it is not evil to seek competent medical care.

This book in itself is the print equivalent of a wonder drug. A remarkably powerful, all-purpose product with enough extra strength to heal every ailment discuss in this book. Techniques are discussed to give solutions to each ailment. Like a wonder drug, the techniques are simple, accessible and virtually risk free

Intelligent, highly trained scientists of unquestionable integrity concluded that each person is biochemically unique. Thus, medicine applied on A and B on the same issue, may have result on A, while B still complain. But perfection, not found in medicine, is found in Jesus.

Once again, prayers are said in the last chapter of the book. If miracles happen in years past, it can still happen in your life. Many who lost hope over their health position, before using this book shall hitherto experience perfect healing of God. Yours is to pray and have faith; then leave the rest to God. If God can perform the under listed miracles in the lives of nation and persons, how can yours be difficult for Him to handle? Imagine: -

Noah built the ark - God flooded the earth

Moses stretched out the rod - God parted the waters.

Joshua marched around the Jericho Walls - God pulled it down

Elisha threw the Stick in the river - God made the iron rises

Naaman dipped himself seven times - God healed him of leprosy

And even so, Jesus commanded the believer; "Lay hands on the sick" - God caused them to recover.

James says; "Elders, anoint any sick with oil, and pray over them the prayer of faith - The Lord shall raise the sick up

The saying doesn't end here. God says, "You do a small thing - I'll do a large thing. What are the large things? They are what you least expect after you receive divine healing. They include among others, testimonies of breakthroughs, mountain built faith, joy, coast expansion, good job etc; and all those things bad health debarred you from attaining.

WHY WORRY?

My last advice here is that you shouldn't worry, since you are not the creator of your life. God didn't create you for the pleasure of your enemy. Therefore, don't worry, for worry is a destroyer of faith. When worry comes, it doesn't come alone, but with fear. When fear enters, faith jumps out. I may not know what you're passing through, I may not know what is ahead of you. What I will tell you is don't worry. Research upon research is carried out on daily basis but with no result. Which type of research? It is research on demon and on worry. In fact, no scientific laboratory can detect the demon of worry, so that it might be killed. The major medicine is *"the medicine of don't worry"*. Really, things may not be working well for you, but because you don't worry, you shall overcome. Many use the 'drug' of don't worry and overcame sickness of fatigue, hypertension, forgetfulness, and many others.

Brethren, why worry? Cast all your care upon Jesus. Cast all your care upon the LORD ALMIGHTY. He is the uncreated creator. No one can challenge him, If within 24hours Satan can attack and destroy the wealth of Job, inflict him with sickness, and at last Job overcame the horrible condition, then I will say don't fear, don't worry. Only see God as having answer to whatever you call problem.

Mind you, anything you place before God, He will jealously guide. See the end of your sickness from the beginning. The source of that sickness shall dry and it shall dry forever. Shout and cry in prayers to God. Forget what people say about you. Don't forget, blind Bartimeaus was shouted down, by the public, when he called on Jesus about his condition.

Alas! As soon as he received his sight, the same public that rejected and look down on him, came rushing with laughter, joy, and with testimonies to congratulate him of the recovery of his sight.

Because, this happened to blind Bartimeaus, because God answered him through Jesus, I say, "you shall recover". Take heart. Today is your day of testimony. Laughter shall fill your mouth. All I will say again is, take heart!

HOW TO USE THE BOOK

This is a multipurpose divine healing prayer book. It can be used to subdue and heal sickness, diseases and infirmities. Also, it can serve as spiritual healing arrow proof and bullet proof against any form of attacks.

The prayers in the book are vomited by the Holy Spirit and should be said during the day or at night for night vigil. It will serve as healing tonic for patients on bed. Such patient can be on bed, sit on bed, or stand on his/her feet as he/she prays the prayers.

If the condition of the patient is critical, whereby he/she cannot read or pray on his/her own, a neighbour or relative can act as an intercessor, praying the prayers in the book on behalf of such patient.

This book should be used on daily basis, until ailment disappears. Let it serve as spiritual companion and tonic against every ailment troubling you. With this book in your hands, there is guarantee of good health, only if you pray, have faith and believe the WORD.

If the sickness persists, ensure you use this book for 7 days night vigil, start from 11 O'clock in the night or 12 O'clock midnight, till 3 O'clock or 4 O'clock A.M. For effectiveness add fasting.

The fast can be from 6 A.M to 12 P.M, 2 P.M or 6 P.M as your strength can take. But, there are ailments that are stubborn, in such situation you can go for a day, two or three days dry fasting, breaking with warm water only at evening times. As you do this, pray fervently. Don't form habit of fasting without praying. Prayer is a must. You must pray and consult your doctor on steps to take. May God be with you, as you receive divine healing today.

Amen

GOOD NEWS!!!

My audiobook is now available, to get one visit acx.com and search **"Tella Olayeri."**

Brethren, to be loaded and reloaded visit: *amazon.com/author/tellaolayeri* for a full spiritual sojourn for my books.

Thanks.

PREVIOUS PUBLICATIONS OF THE AUTHOR

1. <u>100% CONFESSIONS and PROPHECIES to Locate Helpers and helpers to locate you</u>
2. <u>1000 Prayer Points for Children Breakthrough</u>
3. <u>1010 (One Thousand and Ten) DREAMS and Interpretations</u>
4. <u>2000 Dangerous Prayer for First Born</u>
5. <u>365 DREAMS and INTERPRETATIONS</u>
6. <u>430 Prayers to Cancel Bad Dreams and Overcome Witchcraft Powers part one (DREAMS AND YOU Book 1)</u>
7. <u>430 Prayers to Claim Good Dreams and Overcome Witchcraft Powers part two (DREAMS AND YOU Book 2)</u>
8. <u>630 Acidic Prayers: With Missile Prayer for Speedy Breakthrough, Healing and Deliverance</u>
9. <u>650 DREAMS AND INTERPRETATIONS</u>
10. <u>700 Prayers to Clear Unemployment Out of Your Way</u>
11. <u>720 Missile Prayers that Silence Enemies: Prayers that Bring Peace and Rest</u>
12. <u>740 Rocket Prayers that Break Satanic Embargo</u>
13. <u>777 Deliverance Prayers for Healing and Breakthrough</u>
14. <u>800 Deliverance Prayer for Middle Born: Daily Devotional for Teen and Adult</u>

15. <u>800 Deliverance Prayer Points for First Born: Daily Devotional for Teen and Adult</u>

16. <u>800 Deliverance Prayer Points for Last Born: Daily Devotional for Teen and Adult</u>

17. <u>830 Prophecies for the Head: Deliverance Prayer Book for the Brain, Eye, Ear and Mouth</u>

18. <u>Acidic Prayer against Dream Killers</u>

19. <u>Anointing for Eleventh Hour Help: Hope and Help for Your Turbulent Times</u>

20. <u>Atomic Decree that Opens Great Doors</u>

21. <u>Atomic Prayers that Destroy Destiny Killers</u>

22. <u>Atomic Prayers that Destroy Witchcraft Powers and Silence Enemies</u>

23. <u>Biblical Prayer against Sickness and Diseases: Winning the Battle Against Diseases</u>

24. <u>Calling God to Silence Witchcraft Powers: Prayers That Rout Demons</u>

25. <u>Children Deliverance: Power of a Praying Parent</u>

26. <u>COMMAND the DAY: 365 Days of Prayer for Christian that Bring Calm & Peace</u>

27. <u>Command The Night 30 Days Spiritual Manual Prayer Book: A Devotional Prayer Book With 1,200 Violent Prayer Points For Healing Breakthrough and Divine Acceleration</u>

28. <u>Command the Night Against 100 types of Witchcraft Arrows: Powerful Prayers in the War Room</u>

See all at: amazon.com/author/tellaolayeri

Table of Contents

CHAPTER ONE

WHERE IS YOUR HEALTH?

Health is wealth so is said, while sound mind means sound health. Fight and maintain good health in life. Don't waste your life through sickness, disease and infirmity. Pursue and fulfill your destiny. Never allow yourself to be treated like a rain wasted in the forest as a result of ill-health. Sickness is bad to the body while disease kills without notice. Sickness and diseases make people avoid you, for they are open doors to untimely death.

When attacked with disease; no one dare near you as you will be avoided like plague. Just whisper to the ear of your closest friend that you are currently nursing HIV which may soon blow into AIDS. As you tell him; strictly warn him, *"Please don't tell anyone, it is a top secret between me and you"*. Believe it or not, your friend will instantly avoid you. Before you know it, your story shall be a super story all over places. Everyone will avoid you. This is the situation with someone ravaged with sickness and disease. He or she will be avoided by people.

Good health cannot be exchanged for anything. You need it; I equally need good health as well. Good health is a daily crusade affair. It is time for

you to act. It is time to say bye to bad health. It is time to say I shall not die but live and declare the works of the Lord. To achieve this, you shall: -
1. Crush every obstacle assign against your health
2. Call forth healing without prejudice
3. Cry for divine intervention
4. Convert your blood to blood of Jesus
5. Renounce every form of impossibility
6. Contend with dark forces assign against you
7. Lastly believe you shall be healed; and so shall it be.

Health research is carried out on a daily basis, yet it never stop sickness and diseases. Infirmities never seize. We grow and die, while young ones grow to take over. This is the situation in life. Records show that many die young of sickness, diseases and infirmities before their time. Why? It is because there is no permanent solution to health problems. Good health resides with the Lord Almighty. **Samuel F. B. Morse the inventor of The Telegraph in 1844,** had deep thought as he wrote the first message, ***"What has God wrought".*** Here I give the answer. ***"Good things including good health".*** Without good health no human history is complete.

There are specialists all over places, including health sector. They know when heart stop beating death is announced. Hence, they went into research and came out with brilliant ideas and solution of heart problems. In 1966, an American, **Michael Ellis De Bakey** invented **Artificial heart (left vertricle)**. In 1967, **Christian Neethling Barnard,** a South Africa, became **inventor of Human heart transplant.** With these combinations of human efforts, death never die on the surface of earth.

Brethren, may be you don't know how far human beings went into training, education and research to stop death through sickness, diseases and infirmities. They specialise in different fields. Just name it, they are there. We shall mention a few field and their functions now.

1. **Anatomist**:- An anatomist is a person who dissects corpses to know the cause of death.
2. **Cardiologist**:- An expert who study the heart
3. **Cosmetologist**:- A person employed to restore or correct outward appearance.
4. **Dentist**:-A dentist takes care of the teeth.
5. **Dermatologist**:- Expert in the study of skin diseases.
6. **Epidemiologist**:- Expert in the study of spread of diseases .
7. **Gastroenterologist**:- Expert in food recommendation.
8. **Gynecologist**:- Expert in woman and pregnancies
9. **Herbalist**:- Person who use herbs for human solution.

10. **Immunologist**:- Expert in the study of resistance to infection.

11. **Microbiologist:**- Expert in the study of micro-organism

12. **Neurologist**:-Medical expert in the study of nerves.

13. **Obstetrician**:- Medical experts connected with childbirth

14. **Ophthalmologist**:- Expert in the study of the eyes.

15. **Optician**:- Expert who makes and supplies lenses and spectacles.

16. **Orthopaeditrician**:- Expert of surgery dealing with bone deformities and diseases.

17. **Pathologist**:- Expert in the study of diseases.

18. **Pediatrician:**- Physician who specialises in the medicine concerned with children and their illness.

19. **Pharmacist**:- Person professionally qualify to prepare
medicines.

20. **Physician:**- Person qualified to practice both medicine and surgery.

21. **Psychologist**:- Expert in the study of the mind.

22. **Radiotherapist**:- Expert in treatment of disease by means of X-rays.

23. **Surgeon**:- Doctor who performs operations.

24. **Toxicologists**:- Experts in science dealing with the nature and effects of poisons.

25. **Vetenary:**- Expert concerned with the diseases of animals.

Brethren, you can see and read names of experts assign to put things in shape all over places so that sickness, diseases and infirmities find no place in our lives. Yet perfect result cannot be achieved. Our hospital beds are fill, mortuaries are expanding on daily basis for dead bodies. Smiles and laughter are scarce in the faces of people in the hospitals. With these medical wealth of knowledge, sickness and diseases still persist.

Believe me or not, many are sold out to evil creditors in the spirit. Many are sold out to afflictions, sickness, diseases and infirmities. Many dine in bad conditions. Wailing becomes the order of the day as many live in anguish and sorrow. They live in penury because they've spent all they have on sickness. They hardly feed because all is gone. They swim in water of sorrow, baptise in water of sorrow, dine in water of sorrow, drink water of sorrow and what have you. No one sees them without pity saying, *"Who did all these to this fellow"?* This is the situation. But I pray, this shall not be your lot, in the name of Jesus.

I say again, with medical experts and professionals in operation, they are yet to handle situations right. Their best knowledge never give best answer. Volumes of problems pile up on daily basis. Health problems are by day increasing. Medical research is yet to give adequate answer to health problems. Smiles are hardly seen on peoples' faces in hospitals and clinics as "one error or omission lead to untimely death. But then, modem technology has helped to a certain extent. Without it, cries and woes may have risen beyond human imaginations.

Maximum health solution is what we need. It happened before. The Israelites wondered in the wilderness for forty years without epidemic outbreak. They left Egypt with children and women; yet infant mortality rate was below zero level. News of dehydration, cholera, high or low fever, migraine, headache etc were never recorded. Naturally, their shoes and sanders never worn out, neither their cloth torn! What a wonderful result.

There you are! Wonderful results emanate from wonderful source. It is this source that gives wonders of healings. It is this source, that answer health problems with no failure in X-ray reports. There is power behind this. It is Master Jesus, the Prince of Peace. He is the Master Healer, the Healer of healers, the Doctor of doctors, Great Physician of physicians, the King of kings, the Alpha and the Omega.
He is omnipresent, omnipotent and Omniscience.

This Master Jesus, is one who makes impossibility possible. He is the one who can close gate of sudden death fashion against you. He levels up graves dug to consume victims. He is the one that produce answers before you know it. What more? He dries up issue of blood instantly. He raised the dead. He healed the sick. He cast out demons from those afflicted. Withered hands and legs were restored. He opens the eyes of the blind. He cured diverse diseases. He never hesitate to pronounce death upon all sicknesses. Epileptic spirits bowed before Him. Those who were insane regain their minds. Just mention the sickness, diseases or infirmity, Master Jesus is master over them all. He heals without stress. He pronounces the word and it come to pass. The Great healer can heal you. The Mighty Man in battle doesn't fail in his crusade against bad health. Once healed, you're healed. Once cured, you are cured. I say again, whatever he pronounces comes to pass. Master Jesus says, you shall receive your healing today by fire. Amen.

He is calling on you, be desperate to welcome him to your life, He is always at your service. He doesn't die neither does he sleep; He has no holiday neither does he go on sabatical leave. He is twenty-four hours every day ready to answer you. Only, if you call his name. Are you fed up with medical doctors and their reports against your health? Are you at the cross road of health problems? The compass that gives right direction is in his hands. Every health problem harassing you, is nothing but a child play before him. I ask once again, who is this King of Kings? It is Jesus Christ of Nazareth.

Sooner or later you shall open your mouth wide in prayers to this our amiable Prince of Peace, our amiable. Advocate, sitting by the right hand side of the Living God saying, "0 *Lord my Father forgive him his sins and let him be healed"*. And you shall be healed. I say again you shall be healed in the name of Jesus. Amen. Are you doubting? I say again; whether you believe me or not whether you doubt me or not, whether you are a sinner or not, whether you are young or old, you shall receive your healing today by fire in the name of Jesus. I declare it upon you right now, receive your healing, receive your healing, I say receive your healing, in the name of Jesus. Amen.

CHAPTER TWO

JESUS, A HEALING NAME.

The name of Jesus is not ordinary. It is a name that is above every other names, for at the name of Jesus all knee must bow of things in heaven, on earth and below the earth. During and after his ministry on earth demons (the cause of sickness and diseases) bowed before him. At the mention of Jesus' name powers of darkness surrendered. Evil associations scattered. Satan went into hiding, as his efforts and that of his agents wasted before Master Jesus.

Synonymous to Jesus name is divine healing. Jesus never misses word when he said all powers in heaven and on earth has been given unto me. Since peace is his companion he gives peace of mind to people through divine healing. Is your case peculiar? Father Jesus our peculiar Master is at hand to heal you. With His healing, you shall enjoy freedom, damnation of demons and loss of control of demonic powers over you.

The use of his name brings healing. The Bible says, *"And these signs shall follows them that believe, In my name shall they cast out devils; they shall speak with new tongues; They shall take up serpent; and if they drink any deadly thing, it shall not hurt them; they shall lay hands on the sick, and they shall recover" Mark. 16: 17 -18.*

Here, Jesus confirms you can be healed, and can as well
heal people, in His name, because all authority has been given unto him in heaven and on earth. Have faith, your healing is today.

There are wonders and values attached to this name, call Jesus. We have the right to use the name against enemies. These enemies include among others, sickness and diseases and principalities and powers behind such illness. You need to rebuke them using the name of Jesus.

Jesus is all powerful with no exemption as to class. Your sickness, disease or infirmity is a child play game before him. He can heal you. He stands as the Master and the Ruler of the universe. When he rose from the dead, he not only had the keys of death and of hell but he had the very armour in which Satan trusted. As Jesus can put Satan under control, he can equally heal you of ailment. His attention to your situation is what you need. Once you *"arrest"* his attention to your situation all answer to your sickness, disease or infirmity is over. Therefore, stand firm, fear not, believe in his name, the ailment you pass through today, you shall see no more. Poverty and agony which you experience before now, you shall experience no more. Only have believe and faith that God can do it through Jesus Christ of Nazareth.

Why do I have confidence to say this, you might ask. Oh yes, I have confidence to say it because Jesus has defeated the devil, he has defeated all hell, and he stands before the three worlds; heaven, earth and hell as the undisputed victor over man's ancient destroyer, Satan - the author of all ailments. When you believe and call upon Jesus name, he will surely answer you. It is this fresh tremendous victory that made Jesus told his disciples, *"All authority has been given unto me in heaven and on earth"*.

Also, we have the right to use the name in our praises and worship. A reknown man of God in my country Nigeria once said, *"Not all situation and problems one face need to be addressed in prayers alone. Sometimes God need your praises much. He said this through personal contact and experience. He further said, "Some years back, I was called to save a girl who was almost gone. In fact, when I got there, this sister was dead. Her breath had stopped. I now look up, look down, confuse not knowing next step to take. 1 prayed for hours, for her to come back to life, it was as if we were on a wrong track. We pray, pray and pray there was no response. In the midst of confusion, a faint voice came unto me saying; "Praise me and see wonders". Hence, I told everyone around that God wants us to praise Him and get result. Believe me or not, the prayer we did for hours yielded no much result, not until we praised Him. As we praise and flow in the spirit, this girl suddenly sneezed! Everyone was shocked. We never stopped but became "mad", dancing and praising the Lord. Before we knew what was happening, this sister sat down, watched us for a moment, sang the choruses, stood up and join us. The tempo changed. Our "madness" for the Lord increased. There you are brethren, that was how praises, which most people often refer to as common, became the pillar we rested upon to win arrow of sudden death fired against this sister. Praise be to the Lord. Hallelujah.*

The name of Jesus is not a one-way affair. Many opportunities abound in his name. One important fact you must know is this, that the name has been given unto us. The authority he won is delegated to us in that name; all He is today, is in that name, and that name is ours. Jesus was given the Name, that he might give us. Therefore, live and walk in the realm of the supernatural. Walk like a conqueror. Walk out of sickness and diseases. Claim your deliverance today by fire. You are delivered, for no one walk with Jesus and experience defeat from Satan. Your destiny shall not be swallowed by ailment. Agony shall not be your companion. Amen.

All that Jesus was, His name is. He said without missing word, *"And whatsoever ye shall ask in my name, that will I do that the father may be glorified in the Son." John 14:13.* He also said, *Hitherto ye have asked nothing in my name.Ask and yee shall receive that your joy may be made full" John 16:24.* This name will shed blessings, healings and comfort upon human race, and honour and glory to God, the Father.

Today be a mighty army and believer in Christ. After all, we have heard, seen and read of the lame walk, the deaf hear, the blind see: those on the verge of death brought back instantly to health and vigour; but up till now, we have not been able to take permanent place in our privileges and abide where we may enjoy the fullness of this mighty power with divine healing.

As a believer, you. are a disciple of Jesus. What he does, you can equally do; He is not selfish. Address your prayers through the Name, Jesus. In that Name the sick were healed; in that Name demons were cast out; and in that name- the Holy Spirit came upon believers. What does the scriptures says?

In the book of **Colossians 3:17**: We were taught to do all things in that Name, including asking for divine healing.

In the book of **Ephesians 5:20:** We were asked to give thanks always for all things in that Name. Therefore, in every situation give thanks to Him. You shall not die in this situation. The Lord Almighty shall give you instant healing today. Amen

.

In the book of **Corinthian 6:11:** We were washed, sanctified, justified in the Name. Hence, you are washed to be healed. You are sanctified not to experience afflictions in life. Amen.

In the book of **Hebrews 13:15,** Make confessions to His Name. Confess his name upon all situations, and you shall receive answer.

In the book of **James 5:14:** Anoint the sick in the Name of the Lord. By this anointing, all sicknesses shall evaporate out of your life. Diseases shall expire, while infirmities shall vanish by fire.

Don't doubt the use of this name. Many who were held by habits of tobacco, liquor, lust etc. received deliverance by the use of this Name. Many who almost went blind got healed by the power in the name. They threw their reading glass to the dustbin. The blind received sight, those with heart attack got healed, heart disease disappeared, those affected with stroke became whole, those affected with tuberculosis healed. In fact, people with various infirmities received healing at the name of Jesus.

Do you know why God will answer your prayer? Do you know why that sickness. disease or infirmity shall disappear never to re-appear in your life again? The answer is, Jesus won the battle on the cross when he said, *"It is finished"* He meant he has become Master over all problems, over demon and over principalities and power. He is a Master over all sicknesses and diseases. He is a Master over death. There and then. he dramatised it when he was lowered down unto the earth. He wrestled with Satan and his cohorts. He won the battle, He seized the key of death and triumph over death. He seized the key that causes ailment and death as well. He wakes and rise like a triumphant soldier. He marched upon all scorpions and serpents to death. He ascended to heaven as a victor. He became victorious and gave us authority to use His name, so that, we can as well be victorious. No wonder you shall be victorious over your situation today. Amen.

When he gave us Right to use His name, that right meant we are to represent Him, we are acting in His stead, and when we pray in Jesus name, it was as though Jesus Himself was praying. And when Jesus pray, will God listen? Definitely, YES, God will answer His only begotten son. If this is so,

God through Jesus Name shall answer us and blot out our sickness, diseases and infirmities.

This is so because **Jesus** was someone whose **life was full of miracles.** Imagine: -
His **conception** was a miracle
His **birth** was a miracle
His **wisdom** and teaching were miraculous
His **appearances** were miraculous
His **ascension** was a miracle
The day of the **Pentecost** was a miracle
Everything around him and within Him was full of miracles.

Therefore, today you shall experience and receive your divine healing and miracle in the name of Jesus, Hence, I prophesy unto your life, that every disease troubling you shall die. The sickness afflicting you shall die. The infirmity holding you unto ransom shall die, in the name of Jesus.

Today, have a mustard seed of faith so that you receive your healing by fire!

CHAPTER THREE

HEADACHE

Headaches can safely be defined as internal pains in the head. It is a common sickness that need not much introduction. When aches are felt on the head, it is called headache. It is a very rare person indeed who has never experience a headache. About 90 percent of all headaches are classified as muscle contraction, or more commonly, *"tension headaches"*.

Headache is head knocker. The pain is typically generalized all over the head. You may feel dull ache or a sense of not being clearheaded. Most people will describe it as feeling like a bond is wrapped around the head.

The cause of headache is multi various. Scientifically, some people are born with body chemistry that makes them headache prone. The sick history of some family is headache. The complain of both the young and old is headache any time they fall sick. Ask them what killed their grandfather or grandmother it was headache. The little one that died premature death of recent, it was headache that killed him! In such family, headache is their headache.

Really the sickness call headache sometimes is not ordinary. Many are caused by evil arrows, while evil handshakes have resulted to many as well. Also, many die as a result of evil night call as victims shout from sleep with complaints of headache, and before you know it, he has drop dead! This is spiritual attack which we shall address under prayer sessions of this book.

In the practical sense of it, stress contribute to major complaints of headaches this day. When you over stress your brain, headache may follow. Heavy labour under the sun often cause headache as well.

Many people not only get headaches, they get them time and time again. To compound issues many, suffer from migraine which rightfully have uglier reputation than tension headaches. Migraines are part of the vascular headache family and most often strike women. Seventy percent of migraine sufferers are female.

Much pains accompany migraines. It brings severe one sided throbbing pain. At times, the pain occurs on both sides of the head. Often this is accompanied by nausea and vomiting and perhaps tremor and dizziness. Some people also experience premigraine warning symptoms, including blurred vision, *"floating"* visual images, and numbness in an arm or leg.

Funny enough, research has not guarantee diagnose that reveals the kind of headache a patient has. There is no laboratory test that can tell you this patient has migraine or that one has tension. In fact, diagnoses are usually based on the patients' history.

Brethren, regardless of the name you give your headache, tension or migraine, you are the one in best position to recognize what habits and factors you bring on your control to prevent or treat them. So, for a better chance of heading off pain tomorrow, it is good you read the hints below to head off the pain.

HINTS TO HEAD OFF THE PAIN

1. **Take Two, Not Ten.** For that once-or-twice-a-month tension headache, Panadol or one of the many over-the counter anti-inflammatory drugs may work well. All the same, check the use, as over use of these drugs may cause more pain.

2. **Don't Delay.** If you decide to use a particular drug for headache, take it right away; at the beginning of the headache otherwise it may not do you much good.

3. **Exercise to Prevent**. Exercise is useful as a preventive measure. You are releasing stress.

4. **Exercise During. I**f the headache isn't too severe exercise may work to make it better.

5. **Never Exercise if it's Severe**. You'll just make your head hurt more especially if you're suffering a migraine.

6. **Sleep.** A lot of people sleep a headache off and get result of better state of health.

7. **Sleep Straight.** Sleeping in an awkward position or even on your stomach, can cause the muscles in your neck to contract and trigger a headache. Sleeping on your back helps. Try It.

8. **Go Cold.** Nature dictates, some people like the feeling of cold against their foreheads or necks and for them it seems to help.

9. **Heat Up.** To some it is different. They prefer hot showers or putting heat on their necks.

10. **Breathe Deeply.** Deep breathing is a great tension in reliever check it well. You are doing it right if your stomach is moving more than your chest.

11. **Wear a Headband.** This old method of tying a tight cloth around head has some merit to it. The effect is, it will decrease blood flows to the scalp and lessen the throbbing and pounding of a migraine.

12. **Say *"no de cologue"*** It may look strange, strong perfume can set off rnigraine.

13. **Seek Quiet.** Avoid noisy environment. Excessive noise is a common trigger for tension headaches.

14. **Protect Your Eyes.** Bright light - be it from the sun, fluorescent lighting, television or deep motor head lamp can lead to squinting, eyes train, and finally, headache. Sunglasses are a good idea if you're going to be outside. If you're working inside, take some rest-breaks from the computer screen and also wear some type of tinted glasses.

15. **Watch your Caffeine Intake.** Limit yourself to reasonable cups of coffee you take per day. Too much of caffeine will give you a headache

16. **Don't Chew Gum.** The repetitive chewing motion can tighten muscles and bring on a tension headache.

17. **Go Easy on the Salt.** It is unfortunate, high salt intake can trigger migraines, in some people.

18. **Eat on Time.** Skipping or delaying meals can cause headaches two ways. A missed meal can cause muscle tension and, when blood sugar drops from lack of food, the blood vessels of the brain tighten. When you eat again, they expand, leading to headache. Many eat a lot of small meals to keep it in check.

19. **Know your Danger Foods.** There are headache foods. Know one that affects you and stop its consumption.

20. **Say No to Chocolate.** Though it's fattening, it also contains tryramine, a chief suspect in causing headaches, although it is said many young people outgrow this chemical reaction.

21. **Don't go Nuts**. And go easy on aged cheeses. Both contain tyramine.

22. **Don't Smoke and Drive.** You shouldn't smoke, at all. But smoking with the car windows down when you're driving in heavy traffic gives you a double dip of carbon monoxide. This gas appears to adversely affect brain blood flow.

23. **Curtail the Cocktails.** Volume drinks make you hit your head on the rocks too many times. Also, some liquors contain tryramine.

24. **Have a sense of Humor**. Play humour and play down stress.

PRAYER POINTS

1. Stress that leads to headache I overcome you by fire, in the name of Jesus.

2. Headache, I am not for you, disappear in my life in the name of Jesus.

3. Every symptom of headache in my life die, in the name of Jesus.

4. Tensions that invite headache, pack your load and go, in the name of Jesus.

5. I shall experience headache no more, in the name of Jesus.

6. Any power assign to attack me with headache be afflicted with it, in the name of Jesus.

7. My head, I clear you of headache receive deliverance in the name of Jesus.

8. I refuse to be headache prone, in the name of Jesus.

Headache! You shall not be my headache, in the name of Jesus.

9. Comment such as, *"The headache is not ordinary"* shall not be my lot in the name of Jesus.

10. Every evil handshake that causes sickness backfire, in

the name of Jesus.

11. I shall not be victim of hospital, in the name of Jesus.

12. My obituary shall not be announced as a result of what people refer to as *"mere headache"* in the name of Jesus.

13. I shall not shout from sleep to death, in the name of Jesus.

14. Every spiritual attack that leads to untimely death scatter, in the name of Jesus.

15. I shall not labour in vain, in the name of Jesus.

16. I shall not lose my sight as a result of headache, in the name ofJesus.

17. O Lord protect me from sudden death in the name of Jesus.

18. Arrow of sickness backfire, in the name of Jesus.

19. Mr. Tension! die in my life in the name of Jesus.

20. I Shall not be candidate of hospital, in the name of Jesus.

21. Thou Balm of Gilead, heal me today, in the name of Jesus

22. I declare it by fire! I am sick free, in the name of Jesus

23. Symptoms of headache shall not eliminate my family, in the name of Jesus.

24 Headache! You shall not be my headache, in the name of Jesus.

CHAPTER FOUR

DIABETES

Diabetes is the disease of the pancreas in which sugar and starchy foods cannot be properly absorbed. A person with diabetes is at risk of heart disease, kidney disease, atherosclerosis, nerve damage, infection, blindness and slow healing. Diabetes sets in when the matchmaking insulin hormone can't handle sugar molecules.

As a result of body chemistry, each person reacts to diabetes in his own way. This means each person has to be under a doctor's care and constantly monitoring. What is good for patient A may not be good enough for patient B. But the focal point is to maintain blood sugar and blood fat as close to normal levels as possible. A diabetes has three rules cornerstones: nutrition, weight control and exercise. These are the areas of focus to reduce or eliminate diabetes from your body.

WAYS TO KEEP IT UNDER CONTROL
1. **Eat Right Diet**. There is no diet that cut across diabetes patient. Each person's diet should be tailored to fit individual needs and life - styles. Above all, diabetes patients are expected to take great deal of carbohydrate, take little protein, but

cut back fat out of diet as it can cause artery clogging. Also, he should eat food with fiber, such as wheat, barley, oats, legumes, vegetables, and fruit. The benefit of fiber to the body is lower cholesterol levels hence, cut cholesterol intake in form of meat and egg yolks, meat and dairy fats.

2. **Caution Sugar Intake.** The intake of sugar must be considerably limited, mostly when you have low insulin reserves that process your food intakes. See your doctor to give expert advice.

3. **Eat Small Meals More Often.** The diabetic body can handle smaller meals more easily because the smaller the meal, the less insulin is needed to handle the glucose influx from each meal. By this, such less food can be handled by less insulin giving room for more constant blood sugar level needed by the body.

4. **Avoid Fish Oil.** Eating fatty fish is not evil but taking fish oil is not encouraged. Omega - 3 capsules may help present atherosclerosis, another diabetes complication, but too much of it may increase blood glucose level.

5. **Lose Weight.** The first thing a diabetic patient should do is to shed weight. Weight loss is first and foremost of all medications and techniques. They often live a sedentary (get seated while working) life, eat a lot; and as such lead to obesity. By this, all you may need is to diet and exercise to help you lose some weight and get your blood sugar and blood fat back to normal.

6. **Do Exercise**. As a diabetic, you need to do regular exercise to get your arms and legs moving, and your heart pumping. When you do exercise, it will strengthen your heartbeat, helps control blood sugar levels and cut the level of cholesterol in your body. Also, it helps you control your weight, increase your stamina, and let you sleep more soundly. Exercise increases the number of insulin receptors on cell surfaces, therefore find a place to put glucose where it's needed, that is inside the cells. Such exercise may include among others walking, jogging, swimming, rowing or bicycling.

7. **Embrace Walking.** This is by far the safest, least stressful and most productive of all exercises. It improves the efficiency of every unit of insulin taken in or produced by the body. Don't sit down

in a place, learn to walk as exercise, it is the best thing for people with diabetes.

8. **Check With Your Doctor.** It is your doctor that can give adequate advice needed as he study your body chemistry. If your diabetes isn't under control or you have complications, exercise can make it worse. If you are a person with high blood pressure, it also need to be controlled. First, your doctor may want you to take a stress test. He may like to interview you to know and judge the effects of any medication you're taking.

9. **Avoid Damaging Exercise.** There are exercises you need not involve yourself. Avoid such exercise as weight lifting, pushing or pulling heavy objects. If you involve yourself in it, it can raise your blood sugar levels and blood pressure, and can make diabetic eye disease worse.

10.**Take Care Of Your Teeth.** Brush your teeth to make it white and avoid plague and tartar that may find place in your mouth. Since diabetics are much more susceptible to infection they are also more susceptible to gum disease, which is a bacterial infection. Make a visit to your dentist for advise and keep a good health.

11.**Pray it Out.** There is nothing impossible with God. You may have tried all you know yet there is no solution. Take your case to God in prayer. He will solve it.

Now let's pray.

PRAYER POINTS

1. My body system reject diabetes, in the name of Jesus.
2. Every agent of darkness assign to inflict me with diabetes die, in the name of Jesus.
3. Owner of evil load carry your load, in the name of Jesus.
4. Dream attack against my soul die, in the name of Jesus.
5. My body absorb sugar in my body normally, in the name of Jesus.
6. My body chemistry, work fine to my support, in the name of Jesus.
7. Starchy food in my body receive right treatment in my body, in the name of Jesus.

8. Heart disease as a result of diabetes die, in the name of Jesus.

9. Kidney disease as a result of diabetes die, in the name of Jesus

10. Lever damage as a result of diabetes stop by fire, in the name of Jesus.

11. Blindness as a result of diabetes expire, in the name of Jesus.

12. Slow healing in my life I rebuke you, my body recieve accelerated healing, in the name of Jesus.

13. Thou insulin hormone in my body work normal in my body, in the name of Jesus.

14. Diabetes! You shall not kill me, therefore die. in the name of Jesus.

15. Every symptom of diabetes in my body die, in the name of Jesus.

16. Foods that cause diabetes you shall not thirst me to death, in the name of Jesus.

17. Spirit of uncontrolled appetite leave me alone and die, in the name of Jesus.

18. My finances shall not waste as a result of diabetes.

19. O Lord, save me from power of sudden death.

20. I shall not die but live to declare the works of God.

21. Excess sugar in my body, melt by fire and dry up, in the name of Jesus.

CHAPTER FIVE

FATIGUE

Fatigue is a condition of being very tired. It comes in connectivity between you and your body chemistry. Eventual result of it is energy crisis. Fatigue is as a result of energy lost due to in balance of style of living, stress, doing right thing wrong time and in wrong proportion e.g. uncontrolled sexual life.

There was this year my country junior team went for international competition. They played well and got to the finals. And for them to lose the match, *"Sport Coup"* was arranged against them. They fell into the trap. Their opponents knew, fatigue can bring these teams to their knees, the night before the finals, beautiful girls of different sizes and shapes were drafted to the hotel where the young boys were camped.

When they saw free *"bush meat"* (girls), as they are often referred to, they had nice time with them till done. It was as if they played their finals on the bed and scored many goals previous night! They lost much energy in sex before the proper match. When they eventually played their opponents, they performed below expectations. They eventually lost the match, lost the golden cup because they ate their future seeds a night before through sex. Their uncontrolled lost for sex make them tired early in the competition. They lost the match. The reason behind it was nothing but fatigue.

You need your inner engine to perfectly work. You need to conserve your energy for good. Doctors will often tell you, *"get plenty rest, eat a balanced diet, and do exercise"*. This is true but gets more of the hints below to enable you be what you want to be as an energetic person.

HINTS FOR A HIGH - ENERGY LIFE

1. **Warm Up**. In your daily activities learn the habit of having an extra of 15 minutes before you start your day. Get to office on time, rest a little then start off. You start with stamina in you and end well.

2. **Eat Complete Breakfast.** Let your breakfast contain the three components of good breakfast, carbohydrates, proteins and fats. Although you may not like fat, but you can get it in proteins you eat.

3. **Have Focus.** The simple rule is knowing where you are going and know how you get there.

Determine what you intend to do, set goals for the day and pursue it.

4. **Arrest Energy Robbers.** Any interest that will work against your interest should be discourage. Put a halt to whatever will steal your time, energy and thoughts. I fit is a problem on the job resolve it. If relatives are over staying, tell them politely to go.

5. **Tackle One Thing at a Time.** Make lists. Know what to do and where to start. This will make you focus and energetic.

6. **Try Multivitamin.** If you are fond of missing meals, dieting or not eating properly, taking one multivitamin and mineral supplement a day is a good idea. Don't depend on multivitamin all day through, eat properly as this is the source of food nutrition to the body that kills fatigue.

7. **Give Up Smoking.** Smoking is a silent killer. It adversely affects the delivery of oxygen to tissues. The result is fatigue.

8. **Make Exercise an all Day Activity.** Your exercise should be spread, not done once at a

time. Occasional rides of stationary bicycle in office by the executive is an exercise. Walking around during break time is an exercise.

9. **Learn to Delegate.** Don't do all at a time. Give to others what they can do. Supervise and correct their mistakes sooner or later, they shall become master of the art.

10. **Shed Weight.** If you are obese, shed your weight. Obesity brings fatigue in course of time.

11. **Blowout the Candle**. Going to bed late, waking up early tells in the body. Its final result is fatigue.

12. **Avoid Alcohol**. Instead of saying, I will limit it to 1 or 2 bottles; why not stop it out right? It is better you stop what will cause future injury today, than find melater in life.

13. **Eat Big Meal as Lunch.** This is good idea but beware of what you eat. Carbohydrate is a fast burner, eat it. Fats burns slowly, avoid taking it in excess. It will slow you down.

14. **Take Vacation.** Work without play makes Jack a play boy. Whether you are self-employed or working for a company, take your annual leave. It is a way of energy booster. There are cases of people who work 5 to 10 years without going for leave. This is wrong. Have time for yourself.

15. **Divert Your Energy.** Strong emotion is physically and mentally draining. Strong emotions like anger or quarrel should be avoided. It tells in the body.

16. **Colour your Environment.** From research, dark house or dark room brings fatigue. Other colours like red for example, is good for short term, high-energy stimulation, while green is good for eliminating distractions and maintaining focus for long periods of time.

17. **Listen to Music and Good Preaches.** When you listen to whatever and whoever peps you up, you feel alive agile and happy.

18. **Drink Water.** Taking water before major outings, walk or work helps a lot at the end of it

all. The water you consume guard against dehydration.

19. **Avoid Unnecessary Machinations.** Know what you swallow as medicines and their effects. Sleeping pills, for example, are notorious for their next-day hangover effects.

PRAYER POINTS

1. My body receive divine energy, in the name of Jesus.
2. What I lost as a result of fatigue, I receive back in a thousand fold, in the name of Jesus.
3. My pocket shall not lack as a result of fatigue, in the name of Jesus.
4. My nerves receive strength, in the name of Jesus.
5. I shall not be candidate of profitless hard work, in the name of Jesus.
6. I shall not take wrong steps that lead to regrets, in the name of Jesus.
7. Wisdom to capture the day, locate me by fire, in the name of Jesus.
8. My start off shall bring results, in the name of Jesus.

9. My body chemistry receive divine support, in the name of Jesus.
10. O Lord, empower me to move ahead of my contemporaries, in the name of Jesus.
11. I refuse to labour in vain, in the name of Jesus.
12. Owner of evil load, carry your load in the name of Jesus.
13. What I will eat to give me strength, O Lord, provide me, in the name of Jesus.
14. Every energy robber in my life die, in the name of Jesus.
15. Energy crisis die, in the name of Jesus.
16. What I will eat that will kill me O Lord deliver me from it, in the name of Jesus.
17. Spirit of covetousness in my life die, in the name of Jesus.
18. My God shall occupy me with what will boost my energy, in the name of Jesus.
19. Medicine of death assign against me leave my way in the name of Jesus.
20. O Lord, save me from power of sudden death, in the name of Jesus.
21. Every arrow of sorrow fired against me backfire.
22. Any power that wants life difficult for me die, in the name of Jesus.

23. Satanic attachment in my body die, in the name of Jesus.
24. Thou blood in my body receive divine healing, in the name of Jesus.
25. Thou heaven disgrace every satanic load frustrating me, in the name of Jesus.

CHAPTER SIX

KIDNEY PROBLEM

Kidney or renal failure in human being is the malfunctioning of kidney or failure of the kidneys to function properly. A healthy person has two kidneys, and if one of the kidneys is infected with disease or pack up, such a kidney will not function well. However, such person can still live with only one kidney, but there would be a serious problem if he can't pass out urine properly.

When a kidney functions properly, it helps pass out excess water and present unnecessary retention of fluid. The **functioning unit of a kidney** is known as **nephrone,** which is responsible for filtration of fluids and getting rid of all waste products in the body. Hence, if one of the kidneys is bad, the nephrone won't work properly, thereby leading to a person retaining excess fluid. Such fluid becomes a poison to the body. When this happens, the fluid in the body may travel back to the heart and cause congestive heart failure which can lead to death.

There are many causes of kidney problems in the body. They include among others, intake of excessive alcohol which leads to kidney stone, excessive consumption of sugar which leads to diabetes as well, high concentration of salt in foods we eat, fatty foods, inheritance from parents, hitting someone in the abdomen, especially where kidneys are located. This is common among boxers. Also, lackadaisical attitude of people not visiting doctors to ascertain the state of their health, forms major source of kidney problems.

Kidney stone is a form of little crystals of salt and minerals in the kidney. There are several kinds of kidney stones and they hurt. Also, there are a number of strategies for doctors ridding victims of a stone. But then, doctors can't always give guarantee of not having it. Once, a victim has a stone, he is at a somewhat higher risk of getting another. Once your doctor is acquainted with your particular stone, the following tips will help reduce your chances of forming another.

HINTS TO SOLUTION·

1. **Avoid Alcohol.** People should desist from taking excessive alcohol so as to avoid being prone to the disease. It is advisable to stop intake of alcohol completely.

2. **Drink Lots of Fluids.** The single most important preventive measure is to increase water consumption. Water dilutes the urine and help stop prevent high concentrations of those salts and minerals that clump together to form stones.

3. **Beware of Calcium.** Most kidney stones are made of' calcium or calcium products. If your doctor says your last stone was calcium-based, you should be concerned of the calcium you take. Check your calcium-rich foods like milk, cheese or butter. You are doing this to limit and not to eliminate.

4. **Try Magnesium and B6.** It is found that a daily supplement of magnesium curtailed stone occurrence, while vitamin B6 may lower the amount of oxalate in the urine. About 60 percent of all stones are known as calcium oxalate stones. Such oxalate stones won't allow your kidney system work fine.

5. **Eat vitamin A-rich Foods.** Whatever kind of stone you have, vitamin A is necessary to keep the living of the urinary tract in shape and help discourage the formation of future stones. Seek doctor's advice on vitamin A supplements you take,

6. **Stay Active.** It is likely you accumulate lot of calcium in the bloodstream when you are inactive. Activity helps to pull calcium back into the bones, where it belongs. For you to escape kidney stones be active. Get out, take a walk, do little exercise.

7. **Cut Down on Salt**. Always avoid food that has high concentration of salt and fat. Cut down consumption of table salt, picked foods (foods preserved with salt or vinegar) and salty foods.

8. **Listen to doctor.** Doctors often counsel that acute renal failure occurs when the disease are allowed to reach severe stage. Renal failure can be cured through dialysis after which the patient would be placed on certain drugs.

PRAYER POINTS

1. Kidney crisis in my life die, in the name of Jesus.
2. My kidney shall not die of disease, in the name of Jesus.
3. My kidney receive divine healing, in the name of Jesus.
4. Every dream attack upon my life backfire, in the name of Jesus.
5. Every infection in my kidney receive healing, in the name of Jesus.
6. My kidney shall not pack up, in the name of Jesus.
7. Nephrone in my kidney receive life, in the name of Jesus.

8. Every owner of evil load carry your load, in the name of Jesus.
9. Every spiritual ambulance assign for my sake catch fire and burn to ashes, in the name of Jesus.
10. I shall not die but live to declare the works of God, in the name of Jesus.
11. Sudden death! I am not your candidate, therefore disappear, in the name of Jesus.
12. What I will eat that will kill me, O Lord, clear them away from me, in the name of Jesus.
13. Every evil inheritance die, in the name of Jesus.
14. My body system receive healing, in the name of Jesus.
15. Kidney stone in me disappear, in the name of Jesus.
16. O Lord empower me to do right thing at the right time, in the name of Jesus.
17. O Lord give me listening ears to good advice, in the name of Jesus.
18. Power that gives perfect healing locate me by fire, in the name of Jesus.   .
19. Lord Jesus take me to your laboratory and heal me, in the name of Jesus.
20. My Father, my Father, don't leave me in this situation I need your help, in the name of Jesus.

21. Any satanic doctor assign to diagnosis me wrongly disappear from my life, in the name of Jesus.

22. My finances shall not die as a result of sickness, in the name of Jesus.

23. Excess salt in my body expire and disappear, in the name of Jesus.

24. I receive a new kidney, in the name of Jesus.

CHAPTER SEVEN

OBESITY

Part of the food we eat is *"burned"* to make energy. We use this energy to move, breathe, and carry out all our normal daily activities. **The amount of energy present in food is measured in calories.** If a person takes in more calories than his or her body burns up, **the extra calories are stored in form of fat. It is this fat that leads to obesity.**

Obesity is an abnormal accumulation of body fat, usually 20 percent or more over an individual's body weight. Obesity is associated with an increased risk of illness, disability and death. Ideal body weight means the weight a person should be in order to maintain good health. Ideal body weight depends primarily on three factors: gender, age, and height.

Obesity is a matter of degree. There are *four categories*
of Obesity. First, is **Ordinary Obesity.** This person is said to be obesse if his or her body weight is at least 20 percent more than his or her ideal weight. The second is, **Mild Obesity.** A person is said to have mild obesity if he *or* she has a range of 20 to 40 percent overweight. The third is **Moderate Obesity.** A person is said to have this

if he/she has a range of 40 to 100 percent overweight. The fourth is **Morbid Obesity.** A person is said to have this if he/she has more than 100 percent overweight. The erm morbid is used for conditions that can lead to death. It amounts to serious or threatened health problems.

The effect of obesity amounts to serious threath and deadly health problems. These problems include hypertension (high blood ressure), type II diabetes mellitus, coronery (heart disease), infertility, cancer etc. Obesity can also give rise to several other, conditions including: arthritis and other Problems with bones and muscles, such as lower back. pain, hearth burn, high cholestrol levels, menstrual problems, shortness of breath and skin disorders.

WAY OUT

1. **Avoid Fatty Foods.** The best way to prevent obesity is to avoid high intake of fats. Excess of fat in the body leads to obesity. Hence watch fatty foods you eat. Control yourself. The major symptoms of obesity are excessive weight gained and the presence of large amount of fatty tissue.

2. **Have food Diary.** A good way to monitor one's diet is to keep a detailed food diary. This way one will know I exactly how many calories

are consumed in a day and where those calories came from.

3. **Eat enough Carbohydrates.** It is good to choose a diet that will reduce the -risk of gaining weight. Some types of food, such as carbohydrates, are turned into energy more quickly than other types of foods, such as fats. A beneficial diet high in carbohydrates includes cereals, breads, fruits and vegetable.

4. **Choose a Lifestyle.** A person of vigorous exercise is important to burn excess calories. A quiet lifestyle spent watching television will not burn up many calories compared with one that includes swimming, walking or other forms of exercise. Activity is the only way that calories are used up. The more active a person is, the less likely that calories will be converted into fat.

5. **Fight Depressed Mood.** A person may feel depressed or have a low self-image, in response to those feelings, the person may eat more than his or her body really needs. The excess calories are converted to body fat.

6. **Stage of Life.** The stage at which a person first becomes obese can affect his or her ability to lose weight. In childhood, excess calories are

converted into new fat cells. Those fat cells remain in the child's body throughout life. In adulthood, excess calories simply cause existing fat cells to get large. What this means is that obesity in childhood is serious. Research shows that, people who became obese as children have up to five times as many fat cells as those who became obese at adult. Here, parents should counsel children what to eat. Children should learn in their lives the value of a healthful diet and exercise. By controlling their intake of calories and planning activities that will burn them up, the problems of obesity can usually be avoided.

7. **Stop That Drug.** Consumption of certain drugs can also result in obesity. Steroids and antidepressants are examples of such drugs.

8. **Diagnose It.** Doctors can measure body fat with an instrument known as calipers. Calipers are a scissor shaped device used to measure the thickness of a person's flesh at the back of the upper arm. This measurement can be used to tell whether a person has an excess of fatty issue.

9. **Know Your Shape.** Your shape sometimes determine the level of your obesity. Through it, a doctor can know how fat is distributed in the

body and its complications. For example, a person who is *"apple shape"* has a higher risk of cancer, heart disease, and diabetes than someone who is *"pear shaped"*. An *"apple shaped"* person is one whose weight is concentrated around the waist and abdomen. A *"pear-shape"* person is one whose extra weight tends to be around the hips and thighs.

10. **Eat Smaller Units.** Patients should slow down the rate at which they eat during meals. Smaller but frequent meal may serve.

11. **Seek Doctors Counsel.** Going to-doctor for counsel helps to deal with psychological issues that lead to weight gain problems.

12. **Watch that Drug.** Sometimes appetite suppressant drugs are sometimes prescribed to aid in weight loss Appetite suppressants can work on a short term basis, making people to lose weight while they are taking the drugs. But the drugs do not solve the basic problems that lead to obesity. When a person stops taking the drugs, his or her appetite returns. The person once again begins eating too much, and the weight returns. Other side effect includes, dry mouth, headache, constipation, irritability, nausea, nervousness and sweating.

13. **Alternative Treatment.** Most alternative forms of treatment for obesity have problems similar to those of drugs. For example, the Chinese herb Ephedra brings weight - loss on a short term basis. The weight tends to return when use of the herb is discontinued. Consult your doctor, as large amounts of Ephedra can produce a number of side effects such as anxiety irregular heartbeat, heart attack, high blood pressure, insomnia, irritability, nervousness, stroke or death. Also, Diuretic herbs are sometimes recommended for patient.

It is a substance that increase the rate of urine output. As a person produces more urine his or her weight decreases. However, once the herb is discontinued. urine production returns to normal, as does obesity.

14. **Try Natural Remedies.** These include, red pepper and mustard, walnuts and dandelion. For example, red pepper and mustard increase a person metabolic rate at which food is digested. Patients feel thirsty, so he or she is more likely to drink water (which contains no calories) then to eat food. Walnuts, increases the level of brain chemicals that tell a person he or she is no longer hungry.

15. **Do Exercise.** Regular exercise cut down weight. By making exercise a regular part of lifestyle may make you lose weight and to keep

it off. A variety of exercise can be tried so that the patient does not become bored with only one kind of activity

16.**Pray and Fast.** Fasting is good, but don't over eat when you break. By this, your lost weight will be regained fast.

PRAYER POINTS

1. My weight shall not work against me, in the name of Jesus.
2. Arrow of sudden death backfire, in the name of Jesus.
3. Arrow of disability in my life backfire, in the name of Jesus.
4. Every arrow of darkness fired against me backfire, in the name of Jesus.
5. Power of good health locate me by fire, in the name of Jesus.
6. My eating habit receive deliverance, in the name of Jesus.
7. My threatened health receive healing, in the name of Jesus.
8. High blood pressure as a result of obesity die, in the name of Jesus.

9. High cholesterol level as a result of obesity die, in the name of Jesus.

10. Menstrual problems as a result of obesity stop by fire, in the name of Jesus.

11. Sick disorders as a result of obesity disappear, in the name of Jesus.

12. I refuse rejection anywhere I go, in the name of Jesus.

13. Sickness that drain purse in my life die, in the name of Jesus.

14. O Lord, save me from this situation I need your help.

15. Owner of evil load carry your load and die, in the name of Jesus.

16. I shall not reject lifestyle that will favour me, in the name of Jesus.

17. Every depression in my heart die, in the name of Jesus.

18. Power of greatness locate me by fire, in the name of Jesus.

19. Excess fat in my body melt and dry up, in the name of Jesus.

20. Excess water in my body dehydrate by fire, in the name of Jesus.

21. Every coven power expecting my obituary catch fire and roast to ashes in the name of Jesus.

22. Any power assign to mortgage my health die, in the name of Jesus.
23. Spirit of sickness jump out of my life and die, in the name of Jesus.
24. Witchcraft food against me catch fire, in the name of Jesus.

CHAPTER EIGHT

MENOPAUSE

Menopause is the final cessation of the menses at the age of about 50. It begins when the ovaries no longer function. When estrogen secretion slows, then stops, and monthly menstruation becomes irregular, then ceases.

Menopause often create fear in the minds of women, mostly when searching for baby. Non function of ovaries means no baby in sight. It takes miracles for a woman that experiences menopause to put to bed.

During the six months to three years of this cycle of her life, she may feel some of the traditional symptoms of menopause, such as hot flashes and sudden chills, lowered sexual desire, vaginal dryness, emotional upset, and sleeping problems.

No wonder it is often said, when menopause is coming on the way think liberation not liability. Don't look at it as ghost. It is practical and shall surely come. I say, *"think liberation, not liability "*, because during this time you shall experience a sought of freedom!

At this stage you have what is call **PMZ**. What does this stand for? It means **Post-Menopausal**

Zest, a phrase coined by anthropologist **Margaret Mead.** What she meant was that women should seize this stage of life and live it to the fullest. You are free from contraception and pregnancy, and that once-a- month cycle that used to slow you down. This, she says, is freedom.   '

Also, it is a time to explore your environment to its full,
not just as someone who raises children. It is an empowering stage in life. Women should regard it as a cycle time of personal growth and not a decline stage. No wonder menopause is called bittersweet.

HINTS ON GETTING A BETTER OUTLOOK ON LIFE.

1. Design Your Own Zest. Your zest days are close handle with care. It is not fragile but encouraging. Generally, women spend a third of their life post-menopausal. So consider menopause as step forward in life and make a change for the better. It is time you make life an adventure. Find a new hobby. Change careers. Take charge of your health and feel happy!

2. Find Support. Support groups offer reassurance that menopause is a natural cycle. They can offer practical coping techniques discovered as well as sisterly support for new endeavours.

3. Exercise Daily. Walking, Jogging, bicycling, Jumping, Rope dancing, Swimming, or any other daily exercise can relieve a lot of the symptoms of menopause. Such exercise can help prevent or lesson symptoms such as the flashes and night sweats, depression, and other emotional problems, as well as vaginal problems. Stretching exercises are good for flexibility, muscle strengthening, and relaxation. Scientifically, exercise is said to improve psychological health by boosting brain concentrations.

4. Away With that Hot Flashes. Hot flashes are the body's response to lowered estrogen levels. About 80 percent of all women have hot flashes. A typical hot flash last about 2.7 minutes. During a hot flash, your face and upper body feels as if it has been shot into an oven. Your face reddens and you sweat heavily as your skin temperature suddenly rises 7 or 8 degrees. It usually returns in about 30 minutes.

But then, the good news is, many women feel the flash coming just before they actually break into a sweat, so they can prepare for it. The question is, how can you prepare for it? Below, are the how and when.

5. Look Cool. A positive outlook can be an effective daily tool in combating hot flashes. When *you* feel a hot flash coming on, remind yourself of a couple of things that hot flashes are normal, that they don't last long, and that you are able to do something about them. Most times that positive mindset can make the flash more bearable.

6. Learn to Relax. Women who can relax will be in better control. Sit quietly, eyes closed, for a while every day to relax.

7. Control The Triggers. Determine what triggers hot flashes for you, then avoid the triggers. For some women, emotional upset is a trigger. Others may find a hot meal, spicy food, a warm room, or a warm bed will trigger a flash.

8. Go For The Layered Look. Wear sweaters, and vests, then peel a layer off when a hot flash threatens. Add a layer when the hot flash passes because your body temperature actually falls a little below normal and can leave you feeling chilled.

9. Wear Natural Fibers. Synthetic fibers trap heat and perspiration during a hot flash, making this symptom even more uncomfortable. Natural fibers, such as cotton or wool, will give your body more ventilation and keep it cooler by absorbing moisture away from your body and cooling you naturally.

10. Carry a Fan. Buy pretty hand fan and keep it in your purse. You can buy battery powered electronic fan and keep it on your desk. Flip it on as the hot flash again.

11. Eat Small Meals. Rather than load your system three times a day, five or six small meals will help your body regulate temperature more easily.

12. Drink Lots of Water. Always refresh yourself with cool water or juice, especially after exercise. This will keep your body temperature in check.

13. Cut The Caffeine. Caffeine containing beverages stimulate production of the stress hormones that trigger hot flashes.
14. Stop Alcohol. This is another hot flash trigger.

15. Towel Off. Buy small size moist towel. You may want to mop your brow when the heat is most intense or you may want to remove the perspiration after the flash is over.

16. Turn Down the Heat. Heat in any form may trigger hot flashes, leave the window open and avoid hot foods and beverages.

17. Stay Sexy. Women going through menopause who continue to have intercourse on a regular basis (once a week or more) have fewer or no hot flashes compared to women who have sporadic sex.

18. Use Prayer. Apply prayers to kill and destroy problems you might face in respect of menopause appearing before its time or its effects.

Don't worry yourself, just pray. It is either you pray or worry. Since you don't create yourself, why worry? Instead of worry, pray.

PRAYER POINTS

1. Every agenda of darkness to inflict me with infertility scatter, in the name of Jesus.
2. O Lord guide me, and satisfy my soul continually, in the name of Jesus.
3. Satanic dry agent in my body die, in the name of Jesus.
4. Every arrow of disgrace fired against me backfire, in the name of Jesus.
5. My children in heaven cry loud for help and locate me, in the name of Jesus.
6. Thou arrow of darkness fired to scatter my marriage backfire, in the name of Jesus.
7. Lord, heal the wound of my heart, in the name of Jesus.

8. Lord, put an end to my silent suffering, in the name of Jesus.

9. I refuse to be like a stream that goes dry, in the name of Jesus.

10. O Lord, confirm the thought of peace and not of evil you have upon me, in the name of Jesus.

11. I shall start well, and finish well in marriage, in the name of Jesus.

12. My ovaries function well and be normal, in the name of Jesus.

13. Thou Estrogen secretions in my body you shall not slow down or stop, in the name of Jesus.

14. My monthly menstruation become regular, in the name of Jesus.

15. My monthly menstruation, you shall not cease, in the name of Jesus.

16. Thou fear of menopause in my mind die, in the name of Jesus.

17. Symptoms that trigger menopause expire, in the name of Jesus.

18. I recover from sleepless night by fire, in the name of Jesus.

19. Anytime menopause come naturally Satan shall not use it to attack my children, in the name of Jesus.

20. Menopause, you are called Bittersweet, therefore, I claim every sweetness in you at old age, in the name of Jesus.
21. My health shall not degenerate, in the name of Jesus.
22. Hot flashes die, in the name of Jesus.
23. Electric touch from heaven resurrect my menses, in the name of Jesus.
24. Devourer as a result of menopause die, in the name of Jesus.
25. Marital road block in my life scatter, in the name of Jesus.
26. Weeps as a result of menopause clear away, in the name of Jesus.
27. My womb receive divine healing, in the name of Jesus.
28. Dream attack against my life stop by fire, in the name of Jesus.
29. Satanic seal in my body break, in the name of Jesus.

CHAPTER NINE

INFERTILITY

One expects baby after marriage. The purpose of marriage is to produce babies. After the creation of Adam and Eve, *"God bless them and said to them" "Be fruitful and increase in number: fill the earth and subdue it. Rule over the fish of the sea and the birds of the air and over every living creature that moves on the ground". Genesis 1:28*

You can see, God blessed us through our early parents Adam and Eve. But, in the course of time fish of the sea and the birds of the air prosper in fertility while we don't. What must have caused this? What is the way out? For details concerning infertility buy my book titled - **Prayer for the fruit of the womb.**

HINTS TO FOLLOW.

1. Give It A Year. People under 28 often have a wonderful sex life: If there is nothing in your medical history that points to a possible reproductive problem, keep on trying. There is hope. Notice as you get older, naturally fertility decreases a bit. Pray yourself out of spiritual attack. For spiritual support buy my book titled: **Fruit of the womb, and, prayer for pregnant women.**

2. Talk It Out. One of the couple may decide in his / her mind not to be parent any longer and so may frustrate every effort by the other to conceive. Both party should sit down and talk it out. If a need arises see a counselor.

3. Let The Passion Take You. Have passion for sex have passion for baby. Let your heart be at rest. Avoid unnecessary eagerness. Believe it will happen.

4. Ease Up On Your Work Schedule. Your body need rest and not stress. The period of extreme stress is not an ideal time to get pregnant.

5. Stay-on, On Fertility Days. The man -on-top style of intercourse is best for conception. Let the woman remain lying down for 20 minutes after her partner ejaculates. It is advisable for couples to have intercourse on those nights and then fall asleep.

6. Stop Smoking. Cigarettes do impair fertility in men and women. Most men that smoke cigarettes are susceptible to low count sperm than non-smokers. In women it may impair their hormone levels.

PRAYER POINTS

1. Thou coven that close gate of child-bearing against me catch fire and burn to ashes, in the name of Jesus.
2. Thou padlock of darkness fashioned against me, break to pieces, in the name of Jesus.
3. Every prophet of infertility against my marriage die, in the name of Jesus.
4. My marriage hear the word of the Lord, you shall not scatter, in the name of Jesus.
5. Negative scanning result against my womb, you are not my portion, therefore die, in the name of Jesus.
6. Arrow of darkness against my fertility backfire, in the name of Jesus.
7. I receive a new womb, in the name of Jesus.
8. Witchcraft judgment against me scatter, in the name of Jesus.
9. Satanic seal against my womb break, in the name of Jesus.
10. Witchcraft arrow fired against me from my place of birth backfire, in the mime of Jesus.
11. Power to fill the earth and subdue it fall upon me, in the name of Jesus.
12. My womb receive deliverance from the hand of darkness, in the name of Jesus.
13. Reproduction is my right, so I claim it by fire, in the name of Jesus.

14. O Lord, bless me with children and cover my nakedness, in the name of Jesus.
15. Every curse of infertility in my life break in the name of Jesus.
16. Every dream attack against my marriage scatter, in the name of Jesus.
17. Every contrary water and blood in my body dry up, in the name of Jesus.
18. Every arrow of emptiness fired against me backfire, in the name of Jesus.
19. Every power assign to suffocate my hope as a mother die, in the name of Jesus
20. Every seed of infertility in my body die, in the name of Jesus
21. Every arrow of miscarriage fired against me backfire, in the name of Jesus.
22. Every padlock of darkness against my womb break and release me, in the name of Jesus.

CHAPTER TEN

FORGETFULNESS

Forgetfulness is a sickness we often don't notice. Many find it difficult remembering names, phone numbers and important dates. Sometimes many forget how to spell common words. Take the case of this man as an example. A man went out with his car, park it, got into the store, purchase his needs and when he came out; he took public transport, forgetting his car behind. It was not until he arrived home, his wife asked *'where is your car'?* Before he remembered! This is forgetfulness.

While some forgets easily, there are people who are memory experts. They build an iron clad memory and have a super memory brain. Really, some forgetfulness is part of life, but then, you need not wake up one day and forget the name of your spouse!

WAYS TO A BETTER MEMORY
1. Take A Picture. Taking picture of what matters to you, taking part in group photograph helps you remember events.

2. Say It Out Loud. When you talk to yourself in a loud voice on what you need to do or remember, it sticks to your brain for a while.

3. Use An Object As Sign. Tie an object round what you want to remember. It is sign tor physical reminder. This is a very efficient way to remember things.

4. Make Lists. The easiest method is to jot down on paper what you need to remember. By making lists, assure you of remembering what you wrote down on one hand and frees your mind for more important things.

5. Categorize Your Items. When pencil and paper are unavailable, you will have to list things in your head. For example, if you are on your way to a store and you know you need 20 items, you'll probably never remember all 20 unless they are logically grouped. Think five pens, seven books, eight hand bags etc.

6. Chunk. *"Chunking"* is like categorizing, but you do it with numbers. If for instance, you had to remember the numbers 6, 0, 6,3,7,4, I, 5, I, 5. You may have a rough time of it. You can best remember through (606) 374 - 1515. This is quite easier.

7. Make Up A Silly Story. If you've got several items to remember and you are afraid you may forget, you can make up to a tale of it. Let's say you are on your way to purchase, egg, cap, bucket, cup, milk and bread. Tell yourself a story. Place your egg, milk, bread and cup and cap in the bucket. By this you may remember all you need to buy.

8. To Remember Names, Think of Faces. The best way to remember names is to have in your mind a permanent association between the name and the face.

9. Make Name Associations. It is always easier to remember names if you have something to associate the name with. Name of street, an important spot etc. can serve.

10. Look For Important Events. Nothing happens in isolation from other events. Think of a popular thing that will make you remember events.

11. Keep Calm. Stress and anxiety do disrupt memory performance. Your conscience encodes things. Avoid anxiety, it eats that up.

PRAYER POINTS

1. I release my brain from satanic captivity, in the name of Jesus.
2. Every arrow fired against my brain backfire, in the name of Jesus.
3. Brain damage, my brain is not your candidate, therefore expire, in the name of Jesus.
4. My brain receive divine healing, in the name of Jesus.
5. Any evil nail, assign against my brain, pull off, in the name of Jesus.
6. My brain receive deliverance from every works of darkness, in the name of Jesus.
7. I recover my brain from dust bin of life, in the name of Jesus.
8. My Intelligence Quotient **(I.Q.)** be fresh and catching, in the name of Jesus.
9. Every arrow of madness tired against my life backfire, in the name of Jesus.
10. Spirit of the flesh shall not captivate my brain, in the name of Jesus.
11. Padlock of errors and mistakes targeted against my head break to pieces and release me now, in the name of Jesus.
12. As from today I shall not call A for B, or call C for D, in the name of Jesus.
13. By fire, by force, my brain is delivered, in the name of Jesus.

14. Spirit of forgetfulness, leave me alone and die, in the name of Jesus.
15. My brain reject dream attack, in the name of Jesus.
16. Anywhere I go my brain shall measure up to standard, in the name of Jesus.
17. My brain become *'ocean of knowledge',* in the name of Jesus.
18. My brain (my cerebrum, cerebellum- and medulla oblongata) come together for perfection, in the name of Jesus.
19. O Lord, bless me with super memory brain, in the name of Jesus.
20. My brain, I release you from every altar of darkness in the name of Jesus.
21. I shall not be a waste of this generation, in the name of Jesus.
22. Owner of evil load carry your load and die, in the name of Jesus.

CHAPTER ELEVEN

BODY ODOUR

Body odour makes you *'unclean'* among new faces and strangers alike. Body odour can single you out for watch. It develops unnecessary irritation from people. To some, either they perspire not, the odour from their body scents negative attention.

A person with body odour is avoided. They get names they don't bargain for. The simple rule today is, if you want to win friends and influence people don't stink.

From research, there are a quite few ways to take on body odour and come up smelling like a rose.

HINTS TO FOLLOW

1. Scrub Your Body Well. The best way to hold odour at bay is to scrub yourself with soap and water, particularly in those areas of the body that are most likely to smell, such as the armpit sand groin. Body odour is most often caused by a combination of perspiration and bacteria. How often you need to scrub will depend on your individual body chemistry, your activities, your mood, and the time of year. Remember that perspiration glands and bacteria both work night as well as day shifts, which could mean you need to shower both morning and night.

2. Wash More Than Your Body. You need to clean your clothes to match up your bathe. You need a daily change of your shirt or dress to step down any odour that may arise.

3. Choose Natural Fabrics. Natural fabrics such as cotton absorb perspiration better than synthetic materials. The absorbed sweat is then free to evaporate from the fabric.

4. Use Antiperspirants. Commercial deodorants are effective at checking underarm odour in most people. They leave chemicals on the skin that kill off our causing bacteria.

5. Watch What You Eat. The food you eat matters a lot. Extracts of proteins and oils from certain foods and spices remain in your body's execretions and secretions for hours after eating them. This can cause odour. Such foods includes among others, fish, curry and garlic.

6. Keep Calm. Getting sexually excited or feeling anxious and nervious makes one perspire more. In this wise, your anxiety is high. Upsets also increases perspiration. Therefore, learn how to keep calm always.

PRAYER POINTS

1. O Lord, let your divine aroma from heaven envelope my life, in the name of Jesus.
2. O Lord my God, single me out for acceptance anywhere I go, in the name of Jesus.
3. Every unclean spirit assign against me from the pit of hell die, in the name of Jesus.
4. My body become odourless, in the name of Jesus.
5. Every arrow of hatred fired against me backfire, in the name of Jesus.
6. I don't bargain for body odour, therefore, leave me alone and expire, in the name of Jesus.
7. Every symptom causing body odour in me dry up, in the name of Jesus.
8. I reject irritation and replace it with friendliness, in the name of Jesus.
9. I reject bad names as a result of body odour, in the name of Jesus.
10. I shall smell like a rose, and not like a dirt, in the name of Jesus.
11. Thou spirit of poverty in my life die, in the name of Jesus.
12. Every bacteria causing body odour in me die, in the name of Jesus.
13. What I lost as a result of body odour I regain by fire, in the name of Jesus.

14. My past mistakes shall not work against me, in the name of Jesus.
15. I receive freedom from bad odour, in the name of Jesus.
16. I shall not expire before my time, in the name of Jesus.
17. Every mountain facing me as a result of body odour die, in the name of Jesus.
18. River of success and prosperity flow into my life, in the name of Jesus.
19. Odour that magnetise breakthroughs locate me by fire, in the name of Jesus.
20. I convert bad odour to good odour, in the name of Jesus.
21. Favour of God and of men shall locate me, in the name of Jesus.
22. Every bad dream that lead to body odour in me expire, in the name of Jesus.

CHAPTER TWELVE

ARTHRITIS

Arthritis is the commonest disabling disease in the world
that affects the joints more than any other ailment of the joints. Since the joints are very important as they aid easy movement those who suffer arthritis always are rendered helpless once the disease sets in.

Because arthritis is a reaction to cartilage damage, sufferers are always those who are advancing in age, though that does not totally exempt the younger people.

There are more than 200 types of arthritis but the commonest one is **Osteoarthritis.** Really osteoarthritis has commonest one is Osteoarthritis. Really osteoarthritis has a bearing with age. The older you are, the-higher the chances of having articular cartilage damage and the higher the chances of developing osteoarthritis. There are also other things that can damage the articular cartilage sporting activities, infection of the joints, trauma to the joints from sports, road traffic accidents etc.

Osteoarthritis is common among women because the hormone oestrogen which protects them from many diseases, including damage to the articular cartilage, and helps them to maintain their weight becomes absent when they get to' menopause. The protection oestrogen given is then removed. Weight around the waist of women especially African women has bearing on the knee joints. This increases the chance of having arthritis early in life by fat women.

There is a lot you can do on your own, at home, without a lot of expensive equipment or pain or risk. So let's get started.

HELPFUL TIPS FOR ALL TYPES OF ARTHRITIS.

1. **Lose weight, Gain Relief.** Prevention involves a change of lifestyle and early understanding of the damage that can occur in the joints. There is no one magic food or diet that's going to do away with arthritis pain. If you're overweight, lose weight, it will reduce a significant amount of the stress and pain you feel in your spinal column, knees, hips, ankles and feet.

REASON The more overweight you are, the more stress and pressure you place on your joints. This increases the stress on the cartilage, which interferes with the bone, thus increasing the incidence of inflammation, swelling and pain.

1. Solution. Work with your doctor to find a diet that works for you and stick with it.

2. Follow the Movement Rules. There is this moving rules you should follow. Moving hurts, but not moving destroys incorrect moving harms, but intelligent moving heals.

3. Find Relief Through Less Stress. Manage your stress to get relief; know what you can do at a time that will not hurt you later. Don't do all work when you're feeling good. Try to do a little each day, whether you are having a flare-up or not. Learn to relax.

4. Apply Muscle Ointment. Do this at night before going to bed. It relaxes you and gives you a psychological boost as well. There is a new cream in market call URAH produced by Neimeth International Pharmaceutical Plc. It came out with Tronsdermal Glucosomine Cream known as URAH which is absorbed through the skin layers unto the site of pain and. damage, and remains there to work for some time.

5. Try Water Exercise. Water exercise works. It bring relief to people that do it. It is said, your pain will be significantly reduced in the water, and you become much more flexible.

6. Use Ice to Prevent Pain. Have ice in a plastic bag and apply for 15 to 20 minutes on the joints that have been stressed from over use or overwork. Then remove for 10 to 15 minutes. You can repeat for hours at a time. Expect relief to come.

7. Use Heat to Reduce Pain. When joints become hot, swolen, and tender, heat is the best solution, cold would bring pains.

8. Get Off Addictive Drugs. Don't get addicted to drugs. When they are used in ever - increasing amounts, they end up creating many more problems than they solve. Beware of volume of sleeping pills, tranquilizers and narcotic painkillers you use.

9. Fish for Relief. It is observed that patients with rheumatoid arthritis who took fish oil capsules showed improvement in joint tenderness and fatigue. To critics, the active ingredient in fish oil - omega-3 fatty acids has been around in the form of cod-liver for years. Studies have shown that 1 teaspoon per day of cod-liver oil may help alleviate symptoms of reheunmatoid arthritis by providing the body with substantial amounts of vitamin D and A. Vitamin D is important for bone growth, while, vitamin A may have anti-inflammatory effects.

Users should note, both vitamins D and A can be toxic in large amounts, so limit your intake of cod-liver oil to only a teaspoon a day. Also, too much of these vitamins can cause liver damage over time. Please, do consult with your doctor if you think you need fish oil supplements.

10. Boost Your Vitamin C Intake. It is advisable to take vitamin C, as studies have shown that people with rehumatoid arthritis are deficient in vitamin C. Strong doses of it, can bring about regression ofthe disease. See your doctor.

11. Practice Food Avoidance. Results are recorded when patients of roheumatoid arthritis avoid foods from the night shape family and milk. The night shape plant family consists of potatoes, tomatoes, eggplant, tobacco, and all peppers except black pepper. If you take these and your situation get worse avoid them or go for screening with your physician.

12. Cut Back On Vegetable Oil. The benefits of vegetable oil is much, yet caution is given that people with arthritis may be a special case. They may need to minimize their intake of vegetable oils while increasing their intake of oil rich in omega-3 So by this, they should cut back on oil-containing products like salad dressings, fried foods, and margarines. These foods contain. high levels of Omega-6 fatty acids, which can cause inflamation in those with rheumatoid arthritis. It is good to keep the overall level of fat in your diet at less than 30 percent of total calories.

13. Carry on with Carrot Juice. A vegetable-juice fast significantly reduces pain for many patients with rheumatoid arthritis. Carrot juice, celery juice, cabbage juice, or tomato juice can be used.

PRAYER POINTS

1. Every arrow of darkness against my life backfire.
2. Thou disease of arthritis leave me alone and die.
3. My joints (touch them) receive deliverance by fire.
4. I refuse to be rendered useless with sickness, in the name of Jesus.
5. Every symptom of arthritis in my life expire, in the name of Jesus.
6. My lifestyle obey the law of good living, in the name of Jesus.
7. Divine healing from above locate me by fire, in the name of Jesus.
8. Every source of dream attack against my life dry up, in the name of Jesus.
9. I shall not expire before my time, in the name of Jesus.

10. Spirit of leaking pocket assign against me die, in the name of Jesus.
11. Every pain as a result of arthritis die, in Jesus name
12. O Lord, provide me with money to eat right food at right time, in the name of Jesus.
13. Every spiritual obituary organise for my sake scatter.
14. Any evil rope assign to tie my legs in the dream break.
15. My body joints receive deliverance from satanic captivity, in the name of Jesus.
16. Every arrow of sluggishness fired against me from the pit of hell backfire, in the name of Jesus
17. Every power of focal wickedness after my life summersault and die in the name of Jesus.
18. Arrow of motor accident die, in the name of Jesus.
19. Satanic ambulance assign for my sake catch fire and roast to ashes, in the name of Jesus.
20. My body receive power of resurrection, in Jesus name.

CHAPTER THIRTEEN

COLD

Cold is a low temperature when compared with the human body. Cold is a sickness that cut across strata. Everyone succumbs to the common cold. The bravest, the strongest, the sweetest, the smartest, the smallest and the biggest alike are prone to it.

Our virtues matter not to these viruses as they set about reducing us to coughing, sneezing and shivering shadow of our former selves. Cold can be agent of death. It can affect individual as well as group. In Moscow Campaign, Napoleon Bonaparte lost his army of 600,000 who were killed, captured, deserted or died of cold illness leaving only 100,000 remaining. Cold is not friendly, it hurts, leaving cold mark behind.

The real carrier is a virus transmitted through the air. You can catch it when a cold sufferer coughs, sneezes, or blow his nose, sending the virus floating into your path. The question is, can there be remedies to this un-noticed killer of the day? How can you overcome its disorder? Let's see.

REMEDIES TO WIN THE BATTLE.

1. Try Vitamin C. It works in the body as a scavenger, picking up all sorts of trash - including virus trash. When taken, it can shorten the length of a cold from seven days to, may be two or three days. Vitamin C may also cut back on coughing, sneezing and other symptoms. Apart from taking Vitamin C tablet or capsule as prescribed by your doctor, orange, grape fruit and cranbery juices are rich sources of vitamin C.

2. Try Zinc. Sucking on zinc lozenges can cut colds short to an average of four days. Zinc can also dramatically reduce take more than the amount recommended by your doctor. Zinc can be toxic in large doses.

3. Be Positive. Think positive of yourself, it is an imagery technique to combat colds. A positive attitude about your body's ability to heal itself can actually mobilize immune system forces.

4. Rest and Relax. Take rest, not ordinary rest, but extra rest. It enables you to put all your energy into getting well. Such rest can also help you avoid complications like bronchitis and pneumonia.

5. Avoid the Party Lights. When you are sick, parties and other good times can wear you out physically, causing your cold to linger.

6. Take a Walk. Mild exercise improves your circulation, helping your immune system circulate infection fighting antibodies. Take a brisk half-hour walk, but refrain from strenuous exercise which could wear you out.

7. Watch Your Volume Intake. Avoid *"too congesting a diet"* that puts a strain on your body's metabolism. Fatty foods may not haste digestion, eat few of it.

8. Sip Chicken or Pepper Soul. A plate of hot chicken or pepper soup prepared in-house, not necessarily visiting beer parlours, can help unclog your nasal passages. The secretion that comes not when you blow your nose or sneeze, serve a first line of defense in removing germs from your system.

9. Load Up on Liquids. Drink six to eight glasses of water, juice, tea, and other mostly clear liquids daily. This will replace important fluids lost during a cold and help flush out impurities that may be preying and your system.

10. Avoid Smoking. It does two unpleasant things. First, it aggravates a throat that may already feel irritated from a cold. Secondly, it interferes with the infection fighting activity of cilia, the microscopic *"fingers"* that sweep bacteria out of your lungs and throat. Why not avoid what brings no glory to your body? Do so today.

11. Soothe With Saltwater. Wash your irritated throat with a filled glass of warm water and mix 1 teaspoon of salt morning, noon and night, or whenever it hurts most.

12. Get Yourself In Hot Water. Take a steamy shower. Or best, heat a teakettle or pot of water to boiling point on your stove, turn off the flame, cover your head with a towel facing the kettle down, add mentholatum to the water, if you have one, and inhale the steam until it subsides. This also relieves your cough by moistening your dry throat.

13. Apply it Raw. Relieve a nose row from blowing by applying mentholated ointment around and slightly inside your nostrils, this will relieve you.

14. Medicate At Night. Numerous medications for colds are available without prescription. Any medication that have uncomfortable side effects like nausea and drowsiness are recommended to be taken only at nights, since you won't feel the side effects while you're sleeping.

15. Don't Spread Your Germs. Follow the simple rule. When you need to cough, go ahead and cough. When you need to blow your nose, go ahead and blow. But cough and sneeze into disposable tissues instead of setting germs free in the environment. As you do, promptly throw the tissue away and wash your hands.

PRAYER POINTS

1. Every strange cold from the-pit of hell leave me alone and die, in the name of Jesus.
2. Every arrow of sickness fired against me backfire.
3. Every satanic handshake that leads to strange cold expire, in the name of Jesus.
4. Every strange spirit distributing evil cold. I curse you to death, in the name of Jesus.
5. Lord Jesus, lay your hand of healing upon my life
6. I claim normal temperature against cold, in Jesus name.
7. Dream attack against my life scatter, in Jesus name.
8. My soul, escape from the grip of death, in Jesus name.
9. I speak against low temperature, and claim normal temperature, in the name of Jesus.
10. Every virus that cause cold in my life, die in Jesus name.

11. Spirit of cold, you are not parent of sickness in my body therefore, expire by fire in the name of Jesus.
12. Shivering in my life stop by tire, in the name of Jesus.
13. Symptom of cough in my life die, in the name of Jesus.
14. Sneezing, I rebuke you therefore expire by fire, in the name of Jesus.
15. Every agent of death in my life die, in the name of Jesus.
16. Every air pollution attack assigned against me scatter to nothing, in the name of Jesus.
17. I shall not be candidate of hospital in the name of Jesus.
18. My finances shall not be swallowed by sickness, in the name of Jesus.
19. Spirit to relax, rest and receive good health fall upon me, in the name of Jesus.
20. O Lord, provide me with money to buy my needs and eat what is right, in the name of Jesus.
21. I shall not die before my time, in the name of Jesus.

CHAPTER FOURTEEN

VOMITING

Vomiting is the logical conclusion of nausea. Your tummy may have been giving signs of stomach inconsistency. It is saying *'pay attention to me'*. Your tummy's goal is to get rid of whatever you did, that made it sick.

The causes of vomiting are many. It includes among others, sickness. When you are sick, food and or drug taken can be vomited. Intake of wrong food or food that upset body system can lead to vomit. Excess alcohol consumption contributes as well. When you take wrong or harmful tablets, vomiting can set in.

Your primary aim is to avoid vomit. Your goals are to help Mr. Tommy settle down and prevent dehydration

HINTS FOR IT'S PREVENTION.

1. Forget the Stomach Settlers. Most drugs used are not designed to stop vomiting. They are often fit only if the vomiting is related to too much stomach acid. For instance, if you have a stomach ulcer or something you ate is causing irritation. They might work by neutralizing excess acid or soothing irritation.

2. Replace Fluids. When you vomit, you either dehydrate or lose weight. You lose a lot of fluids in vomiting so the best thing you can do is drink fluids to replace those lost. These fluids should be clear liquids; water, weak tea, juices are OK. Fluids like milk or heavy soups may be too much to handle.

3. Replace Important Nutrients. Vomiting flushes out minerals. It is good to take electrolyte drinks. Water is better than nothing, but ideally you should add a couple pinches of salt and sugar to each glass.

4. Sip, Not Slurp. Sipping your fluids in tiny swallow lets your irritated stomach adjust. Sip no more than 1 or 2 ounces at a time.

5. Determine Your Own Timing. Don't rush sips. The less fluid you're sipping at a time, the more often you have to sip. How frequently you take fluids depends on how your stomach react. Once you know you can keep the last sip down, sip some more.

6. Use the Colour Code. If your urine is deep yellow, you're not getting enough fluid. The paler it gets, the better you're doing to prevent dehydration.

7. Go For Warmth. Experts often advise against cold drinks, which shock sensitive stomachs. Room temperature or warm drinks are best.

8. Let the Fizz Out. Tiny bubbles are just what you don't need if you're vomiting. Let your favorite clear carbonated drinks stand until they go flat before you start sipping.

9. Start With Carbohydrates. Sooner or later, vomiting will end. The experts say the best way to start eating again is with a gelatin desert. Jelly like not strong carbohydrate food is recommended way to begin eating after a period of vomiting. Liquid, high in carbohydrates, good tastes are good features of what to take because it will be easy on the stomach. Also, non-buttered toast or crockers are good post vomiting treats.

10. Add a Light Protein. When feeling better, you can move on to a light protein like fish or well cooked meat.

11. Leave Fat for Last. Fat stays in the stomach too long and can thus add to the bloated full feeling. Hence, avoid fatty meats and cream soups.

PRAYER POINTS

1. Arrow of *'eat and vomit whatever you eat'*, backfire, in the name of Jesus.

2. Every evil hand that touch my body to cause me harm wither, in Jesus name.

3. Every sickness that attracts vomiting die, in the name of Jesus.

4. I place heavenly embargo upon every harmful food, in the name of Jesus.

5. Every arrow of dehydration, you shall not catch up with me, in the name of Jesus.

6. O Lord, provide me with money to feed rightly, in Jesus name.

7. I claim good health and not sickness, in Jesus name.

8. Every evil arrow backfire, in the name of Jesus.

9. Evil deposit in my stomach I flush you out with blood of Jesus.

10. I overcome every dream attack, in the name of Jesus.

11. My stomach receive deliverance by fire, in Jesus name.

12. Every power of dream attack against my life backfire.

13. I shall not vomit my virtues away in the dream, in the name of Jesus.

14. Every evil food I eat in the dream die in the name of Jesus.

15. Power of dehydration shall not take over my life in the name of Jesus.

16. I surrender to Jesus not Satan, in the name of Jesus.

17. Divine healing fall upon me in the name of Jesus.

18. Every satanic mathematics against my health scatter in the name of Jesus.

19. My stomach receive healing, in the name of Jesus.

20. Blood of Jesus, soak every food I eat, in Jesus name.

21. I shall not die but live, in the name of Jesus.

22. Divine neutralizer work in me now, in the name of Jesus.

CHAPTER FIFTEEN

SNORING

Snoring is a sleeping disorder. It disturbs sleep of others and is annoying. It reveals when a person sleeps. Both sexes snore, but it is often noticed as one grow. It is hardly found among children but as they grow, the habit reveals itself.

There are heavy snorer and moderate snorer. Men are much more likely to snore than women. Sleep research found that 71 percent of men snored, while only 51 percent of women did. To those who experience snoring, it is not music to the ears at all.

It is an ear sore for singles mostly girls, to snore. It reduces love affections as some men look at such lady as untidy, local or unserious. But the simple truth is, the sound is orchestrated by a wind ensemble located in the back of the throat. The tissue in the upper airway in the back of the throat relaxes during sleep. When you breathe in, it causes this tissue to vibrate, and that effect is very similar to a wind instrument.

WAYS TO HELP STOP THE MUSIC.
1. Go on a Diet. Snoring is frequently related to being overweight. From research, it is found that if a moderate snorer loses weight, the snoring becomes less loud, and in some people it actually

disappears. Most snorers tend to be middle aged, over-weight men. Most women snorers are post menopause. Sliming stops snoring. Just being a little over weight can bring on a problem. The more over weight you are, the more likely it is that your airway will collapse.

2. Ignore the Midnight Spirits. Alcohol before bed makes snoring worse. Don't drink and sleep.

3. Stay Away From Sedatives. Sleeping pills may make you sleep, but they will keep your partner awake. Pills taken relax the tissues around the head and neck will tend to make snoring worse.

4. Put the Cigarette Light Out. Smokers tend to be snorers, so stop smoking.

5. Back Off. When you sleep, sleep on your side, but in case of heavy snorers, they snore in virtually any position. But moderate snorers only snore when they are on their backs.

6. Get On The Ball. Here you need a tennis ball. Sew a tennis ball onto the back of your pejamas. This way when you roll over on your back, you hit this hard object and unconsciously you roll off your back.

7. Have A Fight With Your Pillow. Get rid of it. Pillows only help elevate your snoring level.

8. Raise Your Bed To New Heights. Elevating the bed can help minimize snoring. Do this, put a couple of bricks under the legs at the head of your bed.

9. Blame It On Your Allergies. Sneezing and snoring go together, snoring can develop due to allergies or colds. It is advisable to use a nasal decongestant, especially if your snoring is intermittent and comes during hay fever season.

PRAYER POINTS

1. Sound health be my partner, in the name of Jesus.
2. Every snoring that brings rejection I reject you today, in the name of Jesus.
3. Every attack in the sleep scatter, in the name of Jesus.
4. I refuse to bow to sickness, in the name of Jesus.
5. Snoring, sickness of disgrace leave me alone and die, in the name of Jesus.
6. I shall not breathe the breath of death, in the name of Jesus.
7. I fire back every arrow of darkness fired against me, in the name of Jesus.

8. My inner man receive fire, in the name of Jesus.

9. Every disgrace assign against me scatter, in the name of Jesus.

10. I open a new chapter of sound sleep in my life today, in the name of Jesus.

11. Every satanic nose blockage, expire, in the name of Jesus.

12. Every sleep disorder in my life die, in the name of Jesus.

13. Every hatred my sleep has caused others stop by fire, in the name of Jesus.

14. What I lost as a result of snoring I possess back, in the name of Jesus.

15. I refuse to be a heavy or moderate snorer, in the name of Jesus.

16. O Lord, strengthen my purse to buy right food at right time, in the name of Jesus.

17. Snoring in my life disappear, in the name of Jesus.

18. Power to overcome eating or drinking what leads to snoring fall upon, me in the name of Jesus.

19. I shall not sleep a sleep of death, in the name of Jesus.

20. I shall not serve as negative example, in the name of Jesus.

CHAPTER SIXTEEN

ASTHMA

Asthma is a condition in which the airways (the pathway through which air gets to the lungs for respiration), are hyperactive to various stimuli. Your bronchial airways suddenly contract, you feel a tightness in your chest, you become short of breath, and you cough and wheeze. This is how asthma works.

Different things can trigger off the bouts and periods of hyper-reactivity often call *'attacks'*. One of the things that happen during these attacks is that the airways narrow down and become filled with secretions. All these make it difficult for air to get to the endpoint in the lungs for oxygen to be released into the body. So the person finds it difficult to breath and thus, experiences a choking feeling. Tree, weed, and grass pollens, animal dander, dust mites, and mold are the biggest allergic triggers for asthma.

If you are asthma patient don't panic, no matter what the cause, asthma needn't be a life sentence. There are ways to check it and stop an attack.

HINTS TO STOP AN ATTACK

1. Stay Out Of Smoke-filled Rooms. People with asthma shouldn't smoke, neither should people around asthmatics smoke. If they inhale its smoke, it will affect them.

2. Don't Light A Fire. Throwing another log on the fire, or in the wood store, fuel asthma. If you must make a fire, make sure the room is well ventilated.

3. Stay Out Of The Deep Freeze. Stay indoors when it's cold outside.

4. Buy A Large Scarf. If staying indoors isn't possible, however, make sure you keep your mouth and nose covered when going outdoors, as cold air triggers asthma. But when you have scarf or mask covering your mouths and hose, you end up breathing in warm, humid air.

5. Live In Warm, Dry Place. This is an environment that handles asthma positively to your advantage.

6. Use Auto Air-conditioning Wisely. Air conditioning may be good for asthmatic but not if it is bringing the outside air in. Outside air brings with it pollen, and cool pollinated air is bad for asthma.

7. Watch What You Eat. Eating wrong foods could trigger off asthma. Some of the most common types of foods that trigger asthma are milk, eggs, nuts and sea foods. If you're asthmatic learn which foods can trigger on attack and avoid them.

8. Stay Out Of The Kitchen. Perceiving the foods, you're sensitive to can bring on an attack. If you are allergic to egg, frying it and inhailing the aroma is enough to trigger asthma.
9. Be Salt Sensitive. Researchers discovered that table salt could have a life-threatening effect on your asthma. But the salt wasn't killing people. eating it was. Therefore, control the consumption rate and volume of it.

10. Use Non Aspirin Pain Relievers. For some asthmatics taking aspirin could have life-threatening consequences. Using it could make your asthma worse or even kill you.

11. Use Inhalers Correctly. An inhaler, whether prescribed by a physician or bought over the counter, can bring quick relief to an asthmatic under attack provided it is used correctly.

12. Enlist B6 In The Battle. When a patient use 50 milligrams it is safe but using mega dose may be dangerous. See your doctor.

PRAYER POINTS

1. O Lord, heal every symptom of asthma in my, body in the name of Jesus.
2. Every agent of darkness introducing sickness into my body die, in the name of Jesus.
3. My body, I release you from sickness and diseases, in the name of Jesus.
4. My soul, shall not harbour spirit of sudden death, in the name of Jesus.
5. Every altar of darkness assign against me catch fire, in the name of Jesus.
6. My airways receive strength and not contract in the name of Jesus.
7. O Lord, lay your hand of divine healing upon my life, in the name of Jesus.
8. Owner of evil load, carry your load, in the name of Jesus.
9. Every evil trap assign against me scatter, in the name of Jesus.
10. Fear of sudden death, leave me alone, in the name of Jesus.
11. I shall not die, my enemies shall replace me. in the name of Jesus.
12. Every arrow of sudden death fired against me backfire, in the name of Jesus.
13. I receive divine healing, I am hail and healthy, in the name of Jesus.
14. Every work of darkness against me shall scatter, in the name of Jesus.

15. My father, my father, see to my situation, heal me by fire, in the name of Jesus.
16. Every arrow I receive as a result of this sickness backfire, in the name of Jesus.
17. Blood of Jesus, pollute to death agent of asthma in my body, in the name of Jesus.
18. I shall not shout from sleep to death, in the name of Jesus.
19. I shall laugh at last over ashma, in the name of Jesus.
20. Anything in my environ that triggers asthma die, in the name of Jesus.
21. I am free, and free forever, from power of asthma, in the name of Jesus.
22. I receive complete healing and good health, in the name of Jesus.
23. O Lord, fertilize my pocket and my bank account for your goodness, in the name of Jesus.
24. My body shall not co-operate with works of darkness, in the name of Jesus.
25. Every coven of darkness assign to arrest my soul scatter, in the name of Jesus.
26. My father and my Lord heal me by fire, in the name of Jesus.
27. My breath shall not seize as a result of Asthma, in the name of Jesus.
28. My breath shall praise works of Jesus not works of Satan, in the name of Jesus.

CHAPTER SEVENTEEN

HYPERTENSION (HIGH BLOOD PRESSURE)

Blood pressure (hypertension) is a major health problem. It is one of the most prevalent chronic condition in the nation and one of the major risk factors for heart attack. High blood pressure maintains a weird degree of accuracy for predicting exactly who will get cardiovascular disease after age 65. Hypertension means very high blood pressure that may harm a person's health.

We shall discuss remedies to mild hypertension. Emphasis shall be placed on non-drug therapy. Non drug approach should be the first line of defense to help those with mild hypertension attain good control over their condition.

HINTS TO KEEP IT UNDER CONTROL
1. Watch your Weight. While there are a lot of hypertension who are not fat, obese people tend to have three times as much hypertension as people of normal weight. If you are obese reduce your weight. With relatively minor amounts of weight loss, one can see a measurable fall in blood pressure.

2. Check your Salt Habit. Though there is no yet proven evidence between sodium and high blood pressure. A salt sensitive subset of hypertensive probably exists, and you may be one of them. To know if you're salt sensitive, put yourself on a low - sodium diet and see what effect it has on your blood pressure.

3. Stop Alcohol Consumption. There is a strong connection between alcohol consumption and high blood pressure. It is advisable you stop its consumption. As a Christian you should not patronize it.

4. Avoid Isometrics. Isometric exercises, such as, weight lining must be avoided as it may cause blood pressure to temporarily skyrocket.

5. Try Aerobic Exercise Instead. It has beneficial effect on high blood pressure when you do it with caution. Swimming, walking and bike riding are all good exercises for hypertension. The reason exercise works is that it forces the blood vessels to open up (vasolidatc), and that makes the blood pressure come down. Even though it tends to go back up during exercise, it drops when exercise ends. Then when it goes back up, it doesn't go up as much.

6. Think Vegetarian. Studies have shown that vegetarians have lower blood pressure than the general population. Don't have a misconception of who is a vegetarian. A hemp smoker is not a vegetarian. Those who follow vegetarian diets doesn't smoke, drink or over eat.

7. Measure it Yourself. Do your blood measure reading at home. For anybody who has high blood pressure it is by far the most sensible way to go about monitoring your condition. It can help make you more aware of how diet, exercise, and medications are affecting your blood pressure. It may also help you overcome the *"white coat"* reaction many people experience. The minute they walk in to a doctor's office, they tense up and their pressures rise dramatically.

8. Be a Happy Person. Different emotions play a very specific role in determining how high or low your blood pressure may go. Researcher found that happiness caused systolic blood pressure to drop, while anxiety caused diastolic pressure to rise.

9. Check your Spouse's Pressure too. It is no news that husbands and wives start looking alike after several years of marriage. Researchers have discovered an even stranger phenomenon. The longer two people are married, the more similar their blood pressures become. The time the doctor says your pressure is up, have him check your spouse too.

PRAYER POINTS

1. I cleanse my blood with blood of Jesus.
2. Every mental illness, high blood pressure has caused me, disappear in the name of Jesus.
3. Every suicide spirit in me die, in the name of Jesus.
4. Every arrow of elimination fired against me backfire.
5. I filter sickness in my blood into pit of hell in the name of Jesus.
6. Every satanic blood bank waiting for my blood, catch fire and burn to ashes, in the name of Jesus.
7. I shall not suffer stroke, in the name of Jesus.
8. At old age, confusion and sorrow shall not be my portion in the name of Jesus.
9. O Lord, turn my heart to your heart, in the name of Jesus.
10. Every arrow of hypertension fired against me backfire, in the name of Jesus.
11. Arrow of sudden death backfire, in the name of res us in the name of Jesus.
12. Owner of evil load in my possession, come and carry your load, in the name of Jesus.
13. Bad health shall not swallow my finances, in Jesus name.

14. Oh God, come with your mighty power and expel every symptoms of bad health in my life, in the name of Jesus.
15. Wisdom to excel in life fall upon me, in the name of Jesus.
16. Every injury in my heart receive healing, in the name of Jesus.
17. Every evil seed in my life die, in the name of Jesus.
18. Every troubler of Israel that wants to trouble my soul die, in the name of Jesus.
19. I shall not sleep a sleep of death, in the name of Jesus.
20. My blood, be corrected by the blood of Jesus.
21. Every obituary announcement in the spirit be cancelled, in the name of Jesus.

CHAPTER EIGHTEEN

BACKACHE

Backache simply means pain in the back. Back doctors say the pain comes in two forms, acute and chronic. Acute pain comes on suddenly and intensely. Backache makes you feel unrelaxed. It hurts and pains a lot.

HINTS ON PAIN FREE IDEAS

1. Get Off Your Feet. The first thing you should do is get some bed rest. For the first day or two, keep activity to a minimum.

2. Exercise Through Play Press Up. Press-ups are something like half of a push-up. Lie on the floor on your stomach. Keep your pelvis flat on the floor and push up with your hands, arching your back as you lift your shoulders of fthe floor.

3. Exercise - Move into a Crunch. While on the floor, turn over onto your back and do what is called a crunch sit- up lie flat with both feet on the floor and your knees bent. Cross your arms and rest your hands on your shoulders. Raise your head and shoulders off the floor as high as you can while keeping your lower back on the floor. Hold for one second then repeat.

4. Exercise - Swim on Dry Land. Lie on your stomach on the floor and raise your left arm and your right leg. Hold for one second, and then alternate with your left leg and right arm as if you are swimming. This will extend and strengthen your lower back.

5. Exercise - Get into the Pool. Swimming in a warm pool is a good exercise for acute low back pain. In all, remember - no pain, no gain, no brain. In doing these or any other exercise be careful and know your limit. If the exercise hurts or aggravate you stop doing it; but if you feel fine the day after, or two days, after your exercise, then it is safe to continue, exercising.

6. Kill The Pain on Ice. The best way to cool down an acute flare-up is with ice. It will help reduce swelling and the strain on your hack muscles. Put an ice pack on the site of the pain and massage the spot for 7 to 8 minutes.

7. Try Some Heat Relief. You can switch to heat application after the first day or two of ice. Take a soft towel and put it in a basin of very warm water. Wring it well and apply it in a basin of very warm water. Wring it well and apply it on affected area.

8. Use Heart and Cold. For those who cannot say which is better, apply both methods intermittently.

Do 30 minutes of ice, than 30 minutes of heat, and keep repeating the cycle.

9. Roll Out of Bed. Doctors often advice, when you do have to get out of bed, you roll out, carefully and slowly. But then, let your legs get out of bed first.

10.Lumber Up. Placing cut to size planks under the mattress will help the lumbar lying on top. The lumber end the sagging problem.

11.Take An Aspirin A Day. This can keep back pain away. Using anti - inflammatory drugs helps against pains accompanied by inflammation around the site of the pain.

PRAYER POINTS

1. Every pain attack from the pit of hell backfire, in the name of Jesus.
2. Owner of evil load carry your load in the name of Jesus.
3. I reject sickness I claim divine healing, in the name of Jesus.
4. Thou sickness assign to drain my purse die, in the name of Jesus.
5. My resources shall not fade away as a result of backache, in the name of Jesus.

6. I touch the garment of Jesus, and receive healing, in the name of Jesus.
7. Before sun set I shall receive my healing in the name of Jesus.
8. Every evil handwriting against me be wiped away, in the name of Jesus.
9. I have no case-to answer before Satan, so I am free, in the name of Jesus.
10. By fire, by force, backache shall be a thing of past in my life, in the name of Jesus.
11. My fountain of joy shall not dry, in the name of Jesus.
12. Balm of Gilead heal me today, in the name of Jesus.
13. Every agony of backache disappear in the name of Jesus.
14. Satan your cup is full, disappear in my life, in the name of Jesus.
15. Every satanic instrument assign against my health break to pieces, in the name of Jesus.
16. My back you are not assign for evil load therefore receive freedom, in the name of Jesus.
17. Every arrow of sickness fired against me backfire, in the name of Jesus.
18. Work without pay in my life die, in the name of Jesus.

19. Labour of darkness I reject you by fire, in the name of Jesus.
20. My glory arise and shine, in the name of Jesus.
21. Every occult power working against me die, in the name of Jesus.

CHAPTER NINETEEN

PART B

THE WAY OUT

The way out of sickness is not only by prayer or application of drugs. It is more than this. There are rules to follow. Prayer has guiding rules while drugs have to be prescribed rightly. There are other basic things you must know and do: They are treated briefly below.

1. Be a Child of God. No matter how prayerful you are, not being Born Again, makes your problems re-surface again as avenue is created for Satan to re-enter your life. Satan will surely present his case before God giving reasons why he should stage a counter attack.

2. Have Forgiven Spirit. You must not have any unconfessed or unforgiven sin in your heart, for if you do, demons will laugh at your prayer.

3. Fast. Fasting is essential in prayer and in hygiene. Fasting makes prayer act fast. It suppress mind from evil and awake soul to serve and praise God. All these give room for prayer to act fast. Therefore, incubate yourself with fasting, to fast out your problems.

4. Use Anointing Oil. The application of anointing oil on affected part of your body is biblical. Blessed anointing oil carries fire. It can heal. It can even reveal more than you expect. The book of James 5:14 says, ***"Is any among you sick? Let him call for the elders of the Church; and let them pray over him, anointing him with oil in the name of the Lord"***. Get one today. Let it be blessed by an anointed man *I* woman of God and use it. Note, you are equally call, in as much as you are a Christian. You can equally pray upon your anointing oil and apply it. It all depend on your faith and belief.

5. Be Fast to Repent and Quick to Pray. Repentance without prayer is half measure. Whenever you repent of your sins, crown it with prayer. By this, you are equipped with two edged sword.

6. Check your Dream Life. Your dream life is among other things that dictate your physical. Dream is spiritual but carries weight in the physical. You can receive attack through the dream. For example, when you are injected by a strange person in the dream, it is a bad omen. Having sex with animal in the dream can lead to sickness in the physical. Seeing cat in your dream signifies letter of untimely death in the offing. When led or shown your grave in the dream means death is at hand. Brethren, it is good to know how to interpret dreams to avoid evil. For a better explanation on dreams buy my book titled: **Dictionary of Dreams. It has over 10,000 dreams and interpretations.**

7. Check your Health life. Not all sickness and disease are caused by witches and wizards. Your attitude to life means a lot. A household with unhygienic environment may easily contact disease and sickness. Eating beside un flushed or unprotected toilet can lead to cholera outbreak. Drinking bad water can lead to cholera as well. No witch or wizard attack you. You are the witch or the wizard. The rule is, *"we are what we eat"*. This tells you eat rightly and expect good health. It is good to break through this wall of ignorance and live well.

8. Make Right Confession. Our last confession either destroy or establish our prayer. What I mean is this, beware of what you say after prayer or after a man of God pray for you. When a man of God pray, believe it is established in heaven. Believe, sickness is gone.

Believe all roots of diseases affecting you have withered and die. Have faith, build faith. For example, when a man of God pray for you never say *"Man of God, I want you to keep on praying for me"*. *What you are telling the man of God is this, I know man of God had prayed, but the sickness is yet to go"*. Henceforth, don't entertain fear or doubt. Believe it is done. The statement, nullifies all prayers first uttered by the man of God. For you doubt your faith and invariably doubt God. Always say "I *thank God for answering my prayers"* It shall be established in heaven. Your confession must absolutely agree with the word and if you have prayed in Jesus Name, you should hold fast to your confession. It is easy to destroy the effect of your prayer by negative confession. The Bible says, ***"That they that believe shall lay hands on the sick and they shall recover, and whatsoever ye shall ask in my name, that will I do"***.

9. Let Prayer be your Oxygen. You inhale air to survive. The rule is, *"no air, no life"*. The air you breath is call oxygen. As you make oxygen a *'food"* to survive, make prayer *"food"*, to heal all forms of sickness and diseases. Hence, pray without ceasing.

CHAPTER TWENTY

PRAYER SESSION

All we've seen and adopted as practical guide so far, may not be enough to solve health problem you are facing. Your health problem may be a spiritual attack that needs spiritual counter attack. Arrows fired by power of darkness is an example of this.

It is time to call for healing. It is time to seek it. It is high time to possess it. Who can do it for us? **Who can save us from health calamity? It is Jesus the Son of God. He is sinless and sickless.** He is the one who can do it. He shall do it through our father in heaven, the Almighty God, the I AM that IIAM, the Omnipresent, Omniscience and Omnipotent God. He knows everything and can do everything He can turn impossibility into possibility. He is the Alpha and Omega, knowing the beginning unto the very end. He is the Great Healer.

The Holy Spirit is not left out. He completes the Trinity. He is quiet but active. He is God in the Spirit. We shall continually, call Him into action. He is not left out. Jesus came in physical form, that is why, His name is often used. So when we concentrate using his name much, don't get confuse. You are on the right track.

The first statement of fact is this; in every spiritual battle, Jesus gave us the *'power of Attorney';* legal right to use his name.

Another statement of fact is, all that is invested in His Name, belongs to us, for He gave us the unqualified use of His Name. The book of John 16: 24 clarifies this. ***"Hitherto have ye asked nothing (including good health) in my name: ask, and ye shall receive, that your joy may be full"***. Here, Jesus not only gives you and me the use of His name but He also declares that the prayer, prayed in His Name will receive his special attention. He takes our place, when we pray to God. He is our advocate before God. It is this name; we shall use most in our combat against the unseen forces that surrounds us. Note, Jesus, is one of the TRINITY and the three are One.

CLAIM YOUR RIGHT IN BAPTISM.

Baptizing into the name of the Lord Jesus Christ is richer and full in power. When you baptise into Christ you put on Christ. You are now legally before the world and before heaven a Christian. Baptism in this sense is equivalent to marriage. You are like a wife to Him. When the wife puts on marriage she takes her husband's name and enter into his possessions, and has legal rights in his home. So when as a believer you are baptised into the name of the Lord, you put on the name of the Lord Jesus.

Here, the story changes. You not only put on the name but take your legal right and privileges in Christ. By this, when you are baptised into the name of the Father, it gives you the place of a child and all the privileges of a child, all the inheritance and wealth of the child. Hence, you are baptised into the protection, care and fellowship of the God of the universe.

When you get to prayer session ensure you claim your right so that heaven can visit you; while every foundation of darkness assign against you collapse.

PRAISE AND WORSHIP SONGS

Before we go into prayer proper, a number of songs or worship and praises are written for you to sing. Please forget about the situation you are facing right now. Give thanksgiving unto the Lord through praises, so that gates and windows of heaven may open unto your prayers. Praise Him, so that God can move in His majestic seat in heaven. Praise Him, I say praise Him, so that you can win His favour and mercy concerning your condition. Praise Him, so that you draw His hand down upon you for divine touch and miracles.

SING THE FOLLOWING SONGS OR PICK SONGS OF YOUR CHOICE.

1. The Rock that never fail let me hide in you, in you there is power.
2. Holy Ghost arise in your power
3. What the Lord has done for me
4. Covenant keeping God there is no one like you
5. Darling Jesus, darling Jesus
6. Angels are singing
7. What a mighty God we serve
8. God must be honour
9. Take glory Father, take glory Son
10. Let God arise and my enemies be scattered.

THANKSGIVING·

I thank you O Lord that I am alive today. Many with brief illness passed away within a twinkling of an eye but you never allow mine to be so. To this, I give you glory and honour. My thanks go to you O Lord because in this prayer you shall turn my sickness to healing, my afflictions to liberty, my trials to testimonies, while my sorrow shall turn to joy.

I thank you in advance for the wonderful deliverance I shall experience during and after this prayer. I thank you because you will intervene in my situation and baptise me with peace of mind. Your divine protection is what brings joy to me. I shall receive freedom from my adversaries, my nightmare shall be over. Soonest, I shall experience permanent victory over my illness and share testimonies with people.

With. this prayer, I know you will pour your fresh anointing upon me, to disgrace problems and break yokes holding me captive. The Bible says, *"For now will I break his yoke from off thee, and will burst thy bonds in sunder" Nahum 1:13.* I thank you Lord, for you shall let this come to pass. By this, yokes of infirmities upon me shall break, in the name of Jesus.

I praise you O Lord for accepting my thanksgiving. I praise you because my prayers shall receive answer without delay. Praises shall not seize in my mouth because I know my God shall do it. I will praise, praise and praise you because I know my healing is now.

NOW SING THIS SONG
PRAISE GOD HALLELUYAH
PRAISE GOD AMEN
PRAISE GOD HALLELUYAH
PRAISE GOD AMEN

I praise and give thanks unto you Lord because I know you shall heal me. Your healing brings peace. You added no sorrow unto it, as the Bible clearly said it. *"Then you will go on your way in safety and your foot will not stumble, when you lie down you will not be afraid, when you lie down; your sleep will be sweet". Proverbs 3: 23.* I thank you Lord that my prayers shall bring joy, divine healing and peace of mind. Amen

CONFESSION OF SIN

O Lord I am a sinner before you. Cleanse me of my guilt, for I am loaded with guilt. My romance with sins cause me these. The stubbornness of my heart added fuel to it. Sins led me into captivity of Satan and the punishment is high. I am under the groan of sickness, diseases makes good day in my body.

If only you forgive me O Lord, with time this agony will fade away. Sickness has made friends and relations avoid me. The shame sickness brought I cannot bear anymore, but the root cause is my sin. I say again, if only you forgive me of my sins, I will see your face and you will make me whole.

I know I am reaping the fruit of my sin, for the Bible says, *"A person will reap exactly what he plants. Galatians 6 : 7B.* I regret all the sins I committed ever before now and promise never to go back to it. Have mercy upon me O Lord, *Wash away all my iniquity and cleanse me from my sin". Psalm 51 : 2.* As you forgive me Lord let holiness reign in my life. Let .holiness run through my veins. Let it fill my mouth and actions; -for *"without holiness no one will see the Lord Hebrew 12:14.* I seek your face O Lord for mercy and healing.

I know your healing is perfect, no X-ray can fault it. When you heal, you heal. It is final. When herbalist heal the sickness resurface before you know it. When doctors or physicians heal, it is never a permanent issue. Before you know it, the same complain arise again. But yours is wonderful, supernatural and miraculous. In fact, when you heal it is a permanent issue, unless if one goes back into his / her sinful way again. There and then, the law of holiness is broken and the sickness is invited. But then, I promise O Lord I will not go back - into sin anymore. One thing I will seek from you at this junction Lord is this, protect and guide me. I don't want to dance in the palace of sin any longer. I don't want to walk in the street of sin. In fact, I don't want to speak sin or commit it any longer. Enough is enough.

NOW SING THIS SONG
WHO IS LIKE UNTO THEE O LORD
WHO IS LIKE THEE O LORD
AMONG THE gods WHO IS LIKE THEE
GLORIOUS IN HOLINESS
FEARFUL IN PRAISES
DOING WONDER HALLELUYAH

O Lord let me experience wonders of forgiveness in you. Let your wonders bring me healing, joy and breakthrough. You are the one who can forgive. "There ***is no one like you; you are mighty, and your name is great and powerful" Jeremiah 20 18.*** No one has divine healing power, except you. With you I am in save hands, only forgive my sins and I will survive the sickness.

Satan, you lost outright, my Daddy has forgiven me of my sins. Sickness shall not be my portion any longer. Disease shall find no place in my life. Infirmity shall not be my companion, in the name of Jesus.

Forgive me of my sins Oh Lord, for if you bore my sin, I don't need to bear them. If you bore my sin nature, I don't need to bear it. If you bore my infirmities, I don't need to bear them. For if I bear them it means you die for nothing. And I know it wasn't so. I thank you Lord, as you forgive me my sins. Amen.

PLEAD THE BLOOD OF JESUS

I plead the blood of Jesus upon myself, upon my body and upon my destiny. Blood of Jesus cleanse my body of every sickness and diseases. I wash my body clean with blood of Jesus. Oh heaven cleanse me and let my flesh be like that of a new born baby without stain. I drink the blood of Jesus to cleanse and purge me of any virus, sickness, or disease, inhabited in my body. I drink the blood of Jesus to choke any strange object or deposit in me to death. I drink the blood of Jesus as divine tonic to revive my life for good health. I drink the blood of Jesus to put works of darkness to shame.

Lord Jesus heal my afflicted heart, heal my brain, heal my head, heal my eyes and every part of my body afflicted by Satan. Heal me from the sole of my feet to the top of my head. Let there be soundness in my spirit, soul and body. Heal me of all spiritual and physical sores, spiritual sickness and diseases by your blood. Let death be far from me. Let inconvenience depart from me. Loose and break every bondage holding my health captive by your precious blood. I sooth my life with the blood of Jesus and with oil of God.

I use blood of Jesus as protective power from all evil and all attacks of the devil for, if 1 am under the blood of Jesus Christ the devil cannot do me any harm. The Bible says in Psalm 91:1, ***"He that dwelleth in the secret place of the most High shall abide under the shadow of the Almighty"*** To dwell under the blood of Jesus Christ is equivalent to dwell in the secret place of the Most High. So, I hide and dwell under the blood of Jesus.

I use blood of Jesus as mighty weapon to overcome all Adversaries assign to choke my health life. I use blood of Jesus as a protective sign post upon my body and upon my house lintels. Satan, hear me well, my house is covered with blood of Jesus, while I am covered with blood of Jesus. For it is written, *"Touch not my anointed, and do my prophets no harm". 1 Chronicles 16:22*. Any power assign to attack me shall go blind by the power in the blood of Jesus. Amen

I shall not accept defeat or resign myself to faith. I shall not accept sickness, disease or infirmity as *'the will of God'*, Sickness comes from Satan. And not from God. Hence, I strongly oppose it, I reject it by fire. Blood of Jesus fight for me today. Let Satan see you in me and flee. Let his attack upon me be in vain. Scatter his conspiracy against my health life with your precious blood. Satan, I command you, flee from me! for I am covered with the blood of Jesus.

APPLY HOLY GHOST FIRE

Holy Ghost, take care of my situation, see me through in this warfare prayers. Arrest my heart to fire prayers. Turn me to a bulldozer *"Prayer machine"*. Make me a tireless prayer warrior. Equip my mouth by fire and with fire. Once I pronounce a word or statement let it come to pass. My situation need urgent answer, I need healing.

Holy Ghost Power, go to the root of my problems and heal me. Let your fire burn to ashes every certificate of ill health, certificate of death and certificate of infirmity assign against me. My life is not for sale, therefore kill every messenger of sickness and messenger of death assign to deliver evil message to me from the pit of hell.

Holy Ghost Power, set hedge of fire around me. Build around me mountain of fire, wall of fire, valley of fire and thunder of fire. Let no satanic agent come near me. Let the fire from you heal me both internally and externally. Heal me of every sickness and diseases, I shall not die but live to proclaim the works of God.

Refine my name by fire, refine my body by fire. Save me from sickness and disease that may cut my life short. Send down your fire. Let me receive deliverance from untimely death. Let spirit of sickness and diseases see me and run. Let them flee without looking back. Let their reverse flight led to their death. My father, my father, send down fire.

NOWSING THIS SONG THREE TIMES
SEND DOWN FIRE
THE HOLY GHOST FIRE
SEND DOWN FIRE AGAIN
THE HOLY GHOST FIRE

Holy Ghost Power, I thank you because you are at work. I thank you because you will perfect your role in my life. I glorify your name and majesty, in Jesus name I pray, Amen

CONFESSION OF NEW BIRTH IN CHRIST JESUS

I surrender my life to Christ! I am dead to my sin. I am dead to my old nature. I am dead to all forms of sickness and diseases. They shall not appear again in my life.

I now arise in the fullness of the Almighty God through Jesus Christ of Nazareth. I am free from sins I am free from every form of sickness and diseases, in the name of Jesus. For the Bible says, ***"Surely he took up our infirmities and carried our sorrows yet we considered him stricken by God, smitten by him, and afflicted. But he was pierced for our transgressions, he was crushed for our iniquities; the punishment that brought us peace was upon him, and by his wounds we are healed" Isaiah 53: 4-5.***

Lord Jesus, your resurrection brought freedom from the dominion of sickness. You put demons into chain and shame. You make them redundant. This made me receive liberty from every form of sickness and disease. I arise with Christ from the tomb. My Lord has set me free I am no more captive to sickness, disease and infirmity. I am made whole. Every principalities and powers assign against me shall die. For, I am free and free indeed forever, Amen.

Satan, you can't put me under condemnation by reminding me of my past sins. There is no condemnation upon me, for I am in Christ Jesus. He has dealth with those sins and put them away. I reject their remembrance, 1 reject seeing their photographs, in the name of Jesus.

Satan, you can't impose disease upon me or make sickness my companion. All these, Master Jesus has taken care of. You have no right to bring their photograph around me or frighten me with them. I am free and free indeed. Amen.

Satan, should you attack my body with any sort of sickness or disease, all I have to do is to call my father's attention to the fact, and the disease shall go. This I know for the Bible says, *"By his stripes we are healed"*. Hence, I claim my healing today, in the name of Jesus.

I know by His resurrection I am justified and I do not need to be re-justified. Hence, I am justified to be clean, sanctified, healed and in good health.

I know by His life, I am made alive, and I am alive. By this, I shall not die. No sickness shall kill me. No disease shall kill me. No ailment shall kill me. No infirmity shall kill me. I shall not enter grave before my time. My body shall not decay while I am alive. I am strong in the Lord. No arrow of darkness shall cut me down. I shall not die, in the name of Jesus.

I refuse to confess weakness and failure, doubt and fear upon my situation. Lord Jesus, you are my resurrection you are my healing, you are my life and health, you are my victory. Give me perfect health, for you are my all in all.

CLAIM YOUR RIGHT IN BAPTISM

I am baptised into the name of our Lord Jesus Christ. This baptism represents spiritual marriage between me and Jesus. When a wife puts on marriage she takes her husband's name and enter into his possessions and has legal rights in his home. As I am baptised with the name of our Lord Jesus, I put on His name. I don't only put on the name but take my legal rights and privileges in Christ. As 1 am baptised into his name it gives me the place of a child and all the privileges of a child, all the inheritance and wealth of a child. I am therefore baptised into the protection, care and fellowship of Jesus.

By this baptism, I am joint heir with Jesus and an heir of God. All the mighty victories Jesus won in his death and resurrection are mine. Therefore, I command victory mine. I command every disease troubling me to die. 1 command all sickness in my life to vanish. I command every affliction and infirmity in my life to die, in the name of Jesus.

I receive the fullness of health in Jesus. No sickness or disease shall by no means find way into my life. All the grace that manifested in Christ enwraps me; and 1 am in it. All perfections of health and beauties in Jesus are mine.
I am complete in Jesus.

Lord Jesus, I am into business with you now. We are into business of faith, business of miracle, business of victory, business of legality, business of healing and business of good health. 1 abide under the shadow of your name. Just name the ailment, your name is above it. Hence no sickness or disease shall captivate me. Thou sickness and disease of any form (mention the sickness troubling you), my body is not your candidate, therefore dry up and die, in the name of Jesus. Amen.

Your name is a name of a conqueror and I am baptised into it and bear the name. Hence, I am a conqueror. Satan shall not conquer me by way of ill health. Neither shall he conquer my spouse, children, or household in the name of Jesus. I am for Jesus, an asset of Christ and not of Satan. *"It is no longer I then that live but Christ liveth in me.* "Amen.

BY HIS CRUCIFISSION I AM VICTORIOUS

Lord Jesus, don't forget, when you were crucified you took my place as a sinner. You bore my sins in your body on the tree. You bore my shame that came through my union with Satan. You bore diseases Satan placed on me. You bore my judgement which was mine, because of my union with God's enemy.

When you died, you carried them into the land of forgetfulness and you rose because you put them away. You not only put my sins away but my shame, sickness, diseases and afflictions.

I stand with you and in you, I am free from them all, as you were free when you rose from the dead. Hence, I claim my victory and freedom from every form of disease and sickness.

Lord Jesus, my claims doesn't end here. Your justification is my justification, your righteousness is my righteousness, your health is my health, your freedom from captivity is mine as well. Your freedom, from condemnation is my freedom from condemnation. Your freedom from infirmities also I possess. For in you I enjoy all that you did and all that you are now. With your power, heal me. My situation needs urgent attention. O Lord I say heal me.

Lord Jesus, your name is supernatural, your body is supernatural, your cloth is supernatural. The woman with issue of blood touched you and she received instant healing. Your hand is supernatural, you mould sand from the ground to replace blind eyes. Your mouth is supernatural, you spoke the word, the blind see, the lame walk, little pieces of fish fed the multitude, while good news from your mouth heal the heart of millions. Your word is not past tense, your miracles are not past tense, whoever believe in you still receive healing. No wonder it is said you are the God of yesterday, today and for ever more. O Lord, speak your word upon my life and I will be healed.

Lord Jesus, answer me by fire. Have you lost your power to Satan? The answer is NO. Have you gone out of business of healing? the answer is NO. Has your name replaced by another name? The answer is still CAPITAL NO. Therefore Lord, arise in your power, dramatise your supernatural healing upon my life. I will not close my mouth, I will shout! I need healing! Heal me by fire!

NOW SING THIS SONG TWO TIMES AND PRAY ON.
I AM SERVINGAGOD OF MIRACLES
I KNOW YES I KNOW
I AM SERVING A GOD OF MIRACLES
I KNOW YES I KNOW.

O Lord, you are a God of miracles, I need miracles. Visit me and my household with miracles. I need healing miracles. I need breakthrough miracles. Let people refer to me as Mr. / Miss / Mrs. Miracle. Visit my health life with healing powers. Disgrace sickness out of my life. Let every root of disease in my life die. Thou infirmities in my life, today is your last day therefore die, in the name of Jesus.

O Lord, if you can perform miracles in the past, why can't you perform it in my life today. It was by miracle Joseph was lifted from the prison to palace. He never encountered sickness or down by any form of disease or infirmity. It was by miracle you released the Israelites from bondage in Egypt. Yet when they passed through the wilderness, death record was zero, except when they claimed to be grasshopper. O Lord, I believe in you, I believe in your power. Rescue me from every ailment that placed me in the wilderness of sickness. Lest I forget Lord, the escape of Daniel from Lion's mouth was a miracle. Save me from the mouth of devourers. Sickness is a devourer, disease is a devourer, infirmity is a devourer, every form of ailment are devourers. Hence, let devourers die in my life. Amen

MY DIVINE HEALING IS TODAY

Mr. Sickness, Mr. Disease, Mr. Infirmity, have you forgotten, I am in business with God? Do you forget the miracles and wonders God wrought years back? Do you forget, He can do as in the past? Lest you forget, hear me and hear me well

Noah built the ark - God flooded the earth

Moses stretched out the rod - God parted the waters

Joshua marched around the Jericho wall - God pulled them down

Elisha threw stick in the river - God made the iron Swim

Naaman dipped seven times - God healed his leprosy.

And even so, Jesus command the believer: "Lay hands on the sick" - *God will cause them to recover.*

And James says: *"Elders, anoint any sick with oil, and pray over them the prayer of faith - the Lord shall raise the sick up. "*

My God says, *"You do a small thing - I'll do a large thing. You do a foolish thing - I'll do a wise thing. You do something that only a man can do - I' ll do something that only I (GOD) can do"*
My God is in action. Whatever I say shall come to pass. Whatever I do my God shall accept.

Therefore, I command sickness, disease and infirmity in my body to die in the name of Jesus. Tragedy of untimely death through sickness shall not be my lot. My God, Jehova-Rapha, the healer, shall heal me. His healing power shall sweep through my body. For my God says, *"I will take sickness away from thee .... the ... the number of thy days I will fulfil" Exodus 23: 25, 26.* Hence, I declare perfect healing upon my body, in the name of Jesus. Amen.

POWER OF DARKNESS SHALL MELT AWAY.

Today, I declare war on every form of sickness and take authority over every form of demonic power in charge by the mighty and conquering name of Jesus. My Lord shall transform my health to perfection. Holy Ghost Power shall purge my blood from satanic injection. My God shall do what I ask, for the Bible says, *"Whatsoever ye shall ask in my name, that will I do, that the father may be glorified in the Son" John 14:13.* By this, I shall not experience deafness, heart attack, stroke, high blood pressure migrane, blindness, paralysis, arthritis, fever, headache etc., in the name of Jesus.

Every covenant and power of libation that marries me to sickness and disease shall break. Every covenant and power of evil mark drawing evil into my life shall die. Any incission troubling my soul and health shall die. Every covenant of affliction upon my life shall break. Every mountain speaking woe against my health shall be rolled away. Hence, every sickness pulling me down or standing on my way to attain good health shall die, in the name of Jesus.

NOW SING THIS SONG
**ANY POWER STANDING ON MY WAY
FALL DOWN AND DIE
ANY POWER STANDING ON MY WAY
FALL DOWN AND DIE**

O Lord, breath your renew breathe of life into my body and suffocate' every sickness and disease in me. Let every repercussion of evil handshake die. Let every yoke of bad health die. Let every altar of sickness dedicated against me burn to ashes, in the name of Jesus.

O Lord, heal my bruised heart Blood of Jesus melt every evil deposit in my body. Every power oppressing my spirit die. Every sickness weighing me down die. I touch the helm of the garment of Jesus and receive healing.   I bind and cast out every spirit of sickness in my body. Any cowry power working against my health backfire. Any dark padlock assign against my health break to pieces. Hence, I receive deliverance from every form of attack and ignorance, in the name of Jesus. Amen

MY HEALTH SHALL NOT DETERIORATE.

O Lord, let your healing power take firm root within me. Heal me, of whatever need to be healed, replace in me whatever needs to be replaced, transform in me whatever needs to be transformed. Hence, I come against every disease of the heart, disease of the lung, cancer of the mouth and of the eye, and every form of cancer in the name of Jesus.

Every sickness in me shall clear away. My body is not a temple of sickness but a temple of God. My ears shall not go dumb, neither shall my eyes go blind. Divine clinic from above shall appear in my situation. Direction of bad health and health hazards assign for my sake shall catch fire and burn to ashes. I shall not enrol in the school of sickness. I shall not rush to bank to withdraw in order to cater for sickness. My purse shall not be drained by sickness. You sickness in my body, whether you know it or not, you are a trespasser. Staying in my body makes you a trespasser, feeding in my body makes you a parasite. My body reject you; because you are not accepted as a tenant or landlord of my body. You are an unwanted stranger, therefore walk out of my body. For the Bible says, *"The stranger shall fade away, and be afraid out of their close places" Psalm 18 : 45*. Hence, I paralyse your activities in my body by the fire of the Holy Ghost, and eject you by the blood of Jesus.

NOW SING THIS SONG
THE BLOOD OF JESUS
THE BLOOD OF JESUS SET ME FREE
FROM SIN AND SORROW
THE BLOOD OF JESUS SET ME FREE
THE BLOOD OF JESUS SHALL SET ME FREE
I declare all rusted spiritual pipe in my body to receive healing. Christ of empty tomb, empty me of all forms of sickness and diseases. Roots of sickness in my body dry up. Power of infirmity in my body expire by fire. O Lord revive, redeem and restore my health. Let the plagues that torment the Egyptian of the old be far from me. Let every power assign to torment me be tormented to death. Let your healing descend upon my life by fire.

Lord Jesus, be my Great Physician. Hold me in your alms of healing. Incubate me with fire of healing. Apply your healing oil upon every sick area of my body. Let your anointing of healing penetrate every cell of my body. Let your renew power, renew my health life. Flush out every impurity in my body.

O Lord glue and marry me to good health. Rub me with your palms for total healing. Lord Jesus, you cleanse the temple on that day, cleanse the temple of my life. Let every seed of sickness in my life die. Let every sponsored witchcraft sickness backfire. Let every sponsored witchcraft **infirmity** pursing me die, in the name of Jesus. This, my God shall do, *"For I know "The arm of the Lord is not too short to save, nor his ear too dull to hear" Isaiah 29: 1.*

AT LAST I SHALL LAUGH

At last I am free of sickness and diseases. Bundle of testimonies shall be my portion. I shall laugh over my mockers. My joy shall know no boundary. My testimonies shall bring people to Christ. Miracles shall pursue me about. What I lost I shall recover in thousand folds. I am a candidate of life and not of death. Every messenger of death assign to deliver me letter of death shall not locate me but shall die on their mission. Every claim of death tying me down shall not prosper over my life. Resurrection power of God shall envelope my life. My story shall change. I raise my staff of prayer to kill all manners of sickness and diseases. I receive the miracle of supernatural healing. Hence, as from today, I shall laugh and laugh and laugh to establish my divine healing, in Jesus name I pray. Amen

FINAL THANKSGIVING

O Lord, I thank you for the healing you wrought in my life today. I thank you because all prayers I said shall be sealed in heaven. My healing shall be permanent, for no power of darkness shall rob me of it. In Jesus name I pray, Amen.

SHARE THE GRACE

The grace of our Lord Jesus Christ, the love of God, and the true fellowship of our Lord Jesus

Christ be with me and-my household, for ever and ever, Amen.

Thank you Jesus am grateful
Praise the Lord, Hallelujah.

YOU HAVE BATTLES TO WIN
TRY THESE BOOKS

1. <u>COMMAND THE DAY: DAILY PRAYER BOOK</u>

Each day of the week is loaded with meanings and divine assurance. God did not create each day of the week for the fun of it. Blessings, success, gifts, resources, hopes, portfolios, duties, rights, prophecies, warnings and challenges, are loaded in each day.

Do you know the language, command or decree you can use to claim what belongs to you in each day of the week? Do you know in Christendom, Monday can be equated to one of the days of creation in Genesis chapter one? Do you know creation lasted for six days and God rested on the seventh day? What day of the week can Christian equate as the first day of the week, if we follow Christian calendar? What day can we call day seven?

This book shall give insight to these questions. It shall explain how you can command each day of the week according to creation in the book of Genesis chapter one.

Above all, you shall exercise your right and claim what is hidden in each day of the week.
Check for this in <u>COMMAND THE DAY: DAILY PRAYER BOOK</u>

2. <u>PRAYER TO REMEMBER DREAMS</u>

A lot of people are passing through this spiritual epidemic on a daily basis. Their dream life is epileptic, having no ability to remember all dreams they dream, or sometimes forget everything entirely. This is nothing but spiritual havoc you need to erase from your spiritual record.
The answer to every form of spiritual blackout caused by spiritual erasers is found in, <u>PRAYER TO REMEMBER DREAMS</u>

3. <u>100% CONFESSIONS AND PROPHECIES TO LOCATE HELPERS AND HELPERS TO LOCATE YOU</u>

This is a wonderful book on confessions and prophecies to locate helpers and helpers to locate you. It is a prayer book loaded with over two thousand (2,000) prayer points.

The book unravels how to locate unknown helpers, prayers to arrest mind of helpers and prayers for manifestation after encounter with helpers.

4. <u>ANOINTING FOR ELEVENTH HOUR HELP: HOPE AND HELP FOR YOUR TURBULENT TIMES</u>

This book tells much of what to do at injury hour called eleventh hour. When you read and use this book as prescribed fear shall vanish in your life when pursuing a project, career or contract.

5. <u>PRAYER TO LOCATE HELPERS AND HELPERS TO LOCATE YOU</u>

Our divine helper is God. He created us to be together and be of help to one another. In the midst of no help we lost out, ending our journey in the wilderness.

There are keys assign to open right doors of life. You need right key to locate your helpers. Enough is enough; of suffering in silence.

With this book, you shall locate your helpers while your helpers shall locate you.

6. FIRE FOR FIRE PART ONE: (PRAYER BOOK BOOK 1)

This prayer book is fast at answering spiritual problems. It is a bulldozer prayer book, full of prayers all through. It is highly recommended for night vigil. Testimonies are pouring in daily from users of this book across the world!

7. PRAYER FOR FRUIT OF THE WOMB: EXPECTING MOTHERS

This prayer book is children magnet. By faith and believe in God Almighty, as soon as you use this book open doors to child bearing shall be yours. Amen

8. PRAYER FOR PREGNANT WOMEN: WITH ALL CHRISTIAN NAMES AND MEANINGS

This is a spiritual prayer book loaded with prayers of solution for pregnant women. As soon as you take in, the prayers you shall pray from day one of conception to the day of delivery are written in this book.

9. <u>**WARFARE IN THE OFFICE: PRAYER TO SILENCE TOUGH TIMES IN OFFICE**</u>

It is high time you pray prayers of power must change hands in office. Use this book and liberate yourself from every form of office yoke.

10. <u>**MY MARRIAGE SHALL NOT BREAK: THE SECRET TO LOVE AND MARRIAGE THAT LASTS**</u>

Marriage is corner piece of life, happiness and joy. You need to hold it tight and guide it from wicked intruders and destroyer of homes.

11. <u>**VICTORY OVER SATANIC HOUSE PART ONE: RIDDING YOUR HOME OF SPIRITUAL DARKNESS**</u>

Are you a tenant, Land lord bombarded left and right, front and back by wicked people around you?
With this book you shall be liberated from the hooks of the enemy.

12. <u>**DICTIONARY OF DREAMS: THE DREAM INTERPRETATION**</u>

DICTIONARY WITH SYMBOLS, SIGNS, AND MEANINGS

This is a must book for every home. It gives accurate details to about **10,000 (Ten thousand) dreams and interpretations,** written in alphabetical order for quick reference and easy digestion. The book portrays spiritual revelations with sound prophetic guidelines. It is loaded with Biblical references and violent prayers.
Ask for yours today.

For Further Enquiries Contact
THE AUTHOR
EVANGELIST TELLA OLAYERI
P.O. Box 1872 Shomolu Lagos.
Tel: 08023583168

FROM AUTHOR'S DESK

BEFORE YOU GO

Hello,

Thank you for purchasing this book. Would you consider posting a review about this book? In addition to providing feedback and arousing others into Christ's bosom, reviews can help other customers to know about the book.

Please take a minute to leave a review on this book.

I would appreciate that!

Thank you in advance, for your review and your patronage!!

Feel free to drop us your prayer request. We will join faith with you and God's power will be released in your life and issue in question.

http://tellaolayeri.com/prayerrequest.php

NOTE: You can get all my books from my website http://tellaolayeri.com

GOOD NEWS!!!

My audiobook is now available, to get one visit **acx.com** and search **"Tella Olayeri."**

Brethren, to be loaded and reloaded visit: amazon.com/author/tellaolayeri for a full spiritual sojourn for my books.

Thanks.